Hysterectomy

A
JOHNS
HOPKINS
PRESS
HEALTH BOOK

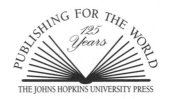

PUBLISHING FOR THE WORLD
125 Years

THE JOHNS HOPKINS UNIVERSITY PRESS

Edward E. Wallach, M.D., is the J. Donald Woodruff Professor of Gynecology in the Department of Gynecology and Obstetrics at the Johns Hopkins University School of Medicine

Esther Eisenberg, M.D., M.P.H., is Professor of Obstetrics and Gynecology and Director of Reproductive Endocrinology and Infertility at the Vanderbilt University School of Medicine

HYSTERECTOMY

Exploring Your Options

Edward E. Wallach, M.D.

Esther Eisenberg, M.D., M.P.H.

THE JOHNS HOPKINS UNIVERSITY PRESS
Baltimore & London

Note to the reader: This book embodies our approach to gynecology *in general.* While we believe and practice its philosophy, we adjust our approach to suit each patient's particular need and each patient's situation. We would not treat any woman without first learning a great deal about her, and so your treatment should not be based solely on what is written here. It must be developed in a dialogue between you and your physician. Our book is written to help you with that dialogue.

The Johns Hopkins University Press
2715 North Charles Street
Baltimore, Maryland 21218-4363
www.press.jhu.edu

Library of Congress Cataloging-in-Publication Data
Wallach, Edward E., 1933–
Hysterectomy : exploring your options / Edward E. Wallach, Esther Eisenberg.
p. cm. — (A Johns Hopkins Press health book)
Includes index.
ISBN 0-8018-7622-2 (hc : alk. paper) — ISBN 0-8018-7623-0 (pbk. : alk. paper)
1. Hysterectomy.   2. Consumer education.   I. Eisenberg, Esther, 1952–   II. Title.
III. Series
RG391.W34 2004
618.1'453—dc21   2003006239

A catalog record for this book is available from the British Library.

Illustrations by Jacqueline Schaffer.

Contents

Preface

Who We Are and Why We Wrote This Book

We became gynecologists because we wanted to help women, an attitude that has been continually reaffirmed through our years of medical practice. We have found that women tend to be open and communicate easily with each other as well as with their physicians. During our training, it also seemed to both of us that obstetricians and gynecologists were upbeat—they were doctors who truly liked what they did. Many women have relationships with their gynecologists that continue over many years, even decades, relationships that encompass the most intimate details of their lives.

In the years since we began our careers, we have seen many changes in the way medical care is provided, but this close, continuing relationship—and the opportunity it allows to help solve a woman's deeply personal problems—is a constant we have observed and valued.

In years past, our chosen field has had its detractors. When Ed began practicing, in the early 1960s, he couldn't help but be aware of a paternalistic and sometimes patronizing approach some of his colleagues had toward their patients. With more feminist sensibilities and an increasingly better educated patient population, this attitude has become much less common.

Esther's earliest experiences as a GYN patient, apprehensive at her first pelvic exam (as so many young women are), convinced her she wanted to do what she could to change medicine. Beginning her practice as an OB-GYN nearly fifteen years after Ed, she knew that some of her medical colleagues viewed those in the profession merely as "baby catchers," with something less than the respect they might have for other medical fields. Recently, however, an interesting combination of politics and technology has turned things around. The women's movement has opened eyes and changed attitudes. And remarkable advances in reproductive technologies have put obstetrics and gynecology at the forefront of medical science.

Which brings us to hysterectomy, the surgical removal of the uterus. Hysterectomy is an important tool for any gynecologist. It is an invaluable treatment for a variety of diseases, a procedure that saves many lives and improves the quality of many others. But an acrimonious discussion often surrounds the subject of hysterectomy, which has become one of the most controversial topics in all of medicine.

As gynecologists, we have been deeply immersed in this discussion and its implications for the women we treat. We believe in the necessity of objectivity—we don't want to scare women out of hysterectomy if it is the best treatment for their condition, but neither do we want to sell it as the cure-all for their problems.

One of the pervasive problems of modern medicine is that doctors may not have enough time, or take enough time, with patients to explain things adequately and answer questions. This failure to communicate leads to many misconceptions, including a common one by physicians that patients understand more than they do. In recent years, for example, Ed has come to realize how many women are ill informed about hysterectomy. He frequently speaks at an annual one-day educational symposium called "A Woman's Journey," at which faculty members of the Johns Hopkins University School of Medicine present information about a range of women's health issues to a large audience composed exclusively of women. His topics are uterine fibroids and endometriosis—not hysterectomy per se, but conditions that sometimes lead to hysterectomy. In the question-and-answer session following his presentations, most of the questions are about hysterectomy. Ed has been struck by the thirst for information on the subject from women who are sophisticated and generally well informed. It has been a revelation to him that the women attending these programs, seeking health information on their own initiative, know so little about hysterectomy—what it entails, when it should be done, how it affects a woman's life (or a couple's life), and what the alternatives might be.

In recent years, most of what those attending the program knew about hysterectomy seemed to come from discussions with friends or relatives and, to a lesser extent, from their own physicians. Even the information from physicians appeared to be fragmented and incomplete. Wasn't there reliable literature on the subject for the lay public?

A search of local bookstores and the public library turned up a number of books about hysterectomy and related subjects, but none seemed to answer satisfactorily the questions Ed had encountered. A number of these books would not serve a woman well as she was making important decisions about her own health care. Titles like *The Ultimate Rape, The Hysterectomy Hoax, You Don't Need a Hysterectomy,* and *No More Hysterectomies* may not provide the objective perspective necessary for this volatile subject.

There was a clear need for a book about hysterectomy for the lay public, particularly for the woman who was contemplating the procedure and for her loved ones. Such a book would provide basic information about the various types of hysterectomy procedures, the reasons for doing a hysterectomy, and the many difficult issues that surround the procedure. It would emphasize the value of hysterectomy but would also express that hysterectomy may be an overused operation and that alternatives sometimes exist. It would reflect the best scientific information currently available as well as personal stories from women who have experienced hysterectomy. That is the book we have tried to write.

Ed and Esther first met and worked together in the 1980s, when Ed was chairman of the Department of Obstetrics and Gynecology at Pennsylvania Hospital in Philadelphia and Esther was a fellow in reproductive endocrinology. Both moved on—Ed to the Johns Hopkins University School of Medicine in Baltimore, to chair the Department of Gynecology and Obstetrics; Esther to Vanderbilt University School of Medicine in Nashville, where she is now director of reproductive endocrinology.

Both of us, in addition to our specialty training in obstetrics and gynecology, have been trained and certified in the subspecialty of reproductive endocrinology and infertility. This means we have devoted our careers to maximizing a woman's reproductive potential and preserving uterine function so that women with fibroids or endometriosis or any of various other gynecologic disorders you will read about in these pages might be treated successfully and have children if that is what they wish. This experience is relevant to our understanding of the hysterectomy issue.

Our years of efforts in helping women become pregnant and give birth have given us a sincere respect for the function of the uterus and its value to a woman. Many women are advised to have a hysterectomy, even when more conservative approaches might be appropriate. We believe that most of the time hysterectomy should be a last-resort treatment option. Still, for thousands of women, hysterectomy has lengthened their lives and provided a better quality of life. Many women speak of "getting their lives back" after hysterectomy.

Our goals are to supply reliable information, dispel misinformation that is based on opinion rather than fact, and provide a reasonable middle ground for discussion. We offer this book as a balanced, comprehensive, accurate, up-to-date, and, we hope, compassionate approach to hysterectomy.

In the pages that follow, we begin, in Part I, by reviewing the anatomy of the uterus and related structures and explaining how the uterus functions normally, especially during the reproductive years. Chapter 2 describes diagnostic tests used to assess the health of a woman's reproductive organs. In Part II, each chapter addresses a specific condition for which a woman might have a hysterectomy, as well as possible therapies for that condition. For most conditions, a number of treatment options should be considered before deciding on hysterectomy.

In Part III, we look more closely at the surgery itself. Chapter 9 describes presurgical examinations and other preparations for a hysterectomy. Chapter 10 covers the issues related to surgery, including differences in length of hospital stay, convalescence period, anesthetic, postoperative recovery, and potential complications. Chapter 11 provides detailed descriptions of the different types of hysterectomies. In Part IV, we examine posthysterectomy issues such as sexuality and reproductive options (Chapter 12) and the possible need for hormone replacement therapy after hysterectomy (Chapter 13). We conclude the book with a final statement of support for our readers, whom we hope we have helped understand and cope with the decisions they may confront in their own "woman's journey."

Note: Because the health care providers we refer to in this book are both male and female, we have alternated gender in pronoun references to health care providers.

Acknowledgments

We thank Jackie Wehmueller for her steadfast role in the publication of this book and also Joanne Wallach, without whose help and encouragement the project would not have been possible. We also acknowledge our patients who shared their stories, which are interspersed within the text.

Hysterectomy

What Is Hysterectomy and What Is the Debate?

Hysterectomy is the name given to the surgical procedure done to remove the uterus. The uterus, also known as a *womb*, is the pear-shaped organ in a woman's pelvis whose primary function is carrying, nurturing, and delivering a baby. The Greek name for this organ is *hystera*, and *ectomy* means surgical removal of any organ—hence the term *hysterectomy*, the surgical removal of the uterus. In ancient times, it was believed that the uterus moved around the body, causing a variety of ailments including hysteria, named for the organ thought to cause it.

Hysterectomies are performed as part of the treatment for a variety of medical conditions, many of which cause pain or abnormal bleeding or interfere with normal function. These conditions include uterine fibroids, pelvic inflammatory disease, endometriosis, adenomyosis, and pelvic relaxation—all of which are discussed in detail in the chapters that follow. Hysterectomies are almost always elective rather than emergency surgery. This means that, except in circumstances such as uterine or cervical cancer, the surgery is performed at the patient's choice—usually with the doctor's recommendation. The elective nature of most hysterectomies is part of what makes the procedure a topic for debate (something we discuss at the end of this chapter).

For nearly as long as hysterectomies have been performed, the uterus was removed through a large incision in the woman's abdomen. Recent advances in medical technology allow less invasive approaches, such as vaginal hysterectomy and laparoscopic hysterectomy (in which tiny instruments are inserted through small incisions in the abdomen). As you will see from the women's stories in this book, there are many reasons and conditions that can lead to hysterectomy—and there are often alternatives to the procedure.

℘ *Adriana was only 22 years old, but her doctor told her she would need a hysterectomy—and soon. "If you want to ever bear a child, get pregnant now," he advised her, "because you are going to need to have your uterus removed." She was devastated but felt fatalistic about her prospects. She had already been diagnosed with endometriosis, adenomyosis, and polyps. Her mother had had a hysterectomy at age 25. But Adriana was so upset at the thought of this surgery at her age that she traveled out of state to get a second opinion from a doctor about whom she had heard good reports.*

The second doctor was horrified. In his view, it would have been a tragedy if Adriana had been persuaded to have a hysterectomy. He knew that there were several treatments far short of hysterectomy that could help her with her various problems. Adriana's medical condition was difficult and would have to be followed closely, but she was also a healthy woman who had received dubious medical advice.

℘ *As she approached her fifties, Helena finally decided that she no longer wanted to put up with the painful menstrual periods and heavy bleeding she had endured all her adult life. For years her doctors had urged her to get a hysterectomy to treat definitively her large and numerous fibroid tumors— fibroids that caused bleeding so heavy it left her anemic, drained of energy, and feeling faint; fibroids that had grown back after myomectomy (surgical removal of just the fibroid) and that had not responded to medications. She worried, as she had for years, about what the surgery would mean for her as a woman, how it would affect her aging, how she would feel afterward. Suppose something more than a diseased anatomic structure—her fibroid-ridden uterus—was lost?*

"You're going to feel better than you have in a long time," her doctor had predicted. Finally, Helena's declining quality of life made her decide in favor of the procedure she had resisted for so long. Her doctor was right. As she healed from the abdominal incision, she felt "fantastic," stronger and healthier than she could remember. She was a new person with a new life, and she couldn't help wondering whether she had cheated herself of years of feeling well by delaying the operation for so long.

Adriana and Helena represent two opposite ends of the hysterectomy discussion: the woman who is advised to have an unnecessary hysterectomy and the woman who delays having one because of fear and misinformation about how it will affect her. Many, many women who have experienced abnormal bleeding and pain at various points in their lives and have sought relief from gynecologic problems can relate to their experiences.

Numerous treatments are available for most gynecologic conditions, and the best course to take is not always obvious. There are risks and benefits to weigh and decisions to make. There are no hard-and-fast rules in the hysterectomy decision. Women seeking second opinions— which we recommend for anyone who is not completely comfortable with her doctor's recommendation—are likely to encounter a range of views. Practices vary greatly, from one region of the country to another and even from doctor to doctor.

THE NUMBERS

More than one-fifth, or 20 percent, of all American women have had a hysterectomy. It is the second most common major surgical procedure performed on women in the United States, second only to cesarean section. About 600,000 hysterectomies are performed each year in this country, which amounts to about 4.1 hysterectomies per 1,000 women. The annual financial cost for this procedure in the United States is estimated at more than $5 billion, but the physical and emotional costs must also be considered.

Current statistics indicate that fewer hysterectomies are being performed. Absolute numbers show one part of this picture—in 1975, for example, 724,000 hysterectomies were performed in the United States. But an even more telling figure is the rate of hysterectomy per 1,000 women, because this figure takes into consideration the increase in the number of American women. The downward trend in that rate has been clear and consistent: in 1975, 8.6 hysterectomies were performed per 1,000 women; in 1980, 7.1; in 1985, 6.9; in 1990, 5.8; in 1995, 5.5; and in 1999, 5.5. Similar declines have been noted in Canada and Great Britain. For the past few years, the rate of hysterectomies has leveled off somewhat, decreasing more slowly than in previous years. But it is likely that new, less invasive surgical approaches such as endometrial ablation and uterine artery embolization (both of which are discussed in the chapters that follow) will lead to further reductions in the hysterectomy rate in the future.

Many women have hysterectomies in the prime of their life—the median age is 40.9 years. Women are most likely to have a hysterectomy between the ages of 35 and 55. Several other statistics highlight how common this procedure is and how often it is performed on relatively young women:

- 20 percent of all women have had a hysterectomy by age 40
- More than 30 percent of women in the United States will have had a hysterectomy by the time they reach 60 years of age
- 39 percent of women have had a hysterectomy by age 65
- The highest rate of hysterectomy is in women aged 40 to 44 years; each year 12 of every 1,000 women this age have a hysterectomy—nearly triple the overall rate

Within the United States there is considerable regional variation in hysterectomy rates and in a woman's age when she has one. This difference is a consequence of a number of factors: cost-containment measures and their variation from state to state; regional differences in medical practice and professional attitudes; recognition of newer options to treat conditions for which hysterectomy has traditionally been used; differences in genetic makeup of different populations; regional variations in patient knowledge and preferences; and pressures by various interest groups. Professional uncertainty regarding difficulties in diagnosis, knowledge of outcome, and alternative treatments is also key in explaining these variations. Then there is the "consumer factor"—patients who lack accurate, understandable information about hysterectomy and its alternatives and patients who exert pressure on their physicians to perform (or not to perform) a hysterectomy also influence how many hysterectomies are done.

The highest annual hysterectomy rates are seen in the South—6.8 per 1,000 women. The lowest hysterectomy rates are in the Northeast, with an average annual rate of 3.9 hysterectomies per 1,000 women. Women in the South are also significantly younger at the time of hysterectomy, compared with those in other regions of the United States. Regionally, the average age at the time of hysterectomy is:

- 47.7 years old for women living in the Northeast
- 44.5 years in the Midwest
- 44.0 years in the West
- 41.6 years in the South

What do these numbers mean to you, the woman who is making a decision about having a hysterectomy? As we have seen, a variety of factors account for the regional differences in hysterectomy rates—different cultural approaches to medical care in general, different genetic patterns in the population, different approaches in medical education leading to different preferences among doctors, and different patient preferences. Even within a geographic region, physicians in private practice in rural areas may practice differently from physicians in an urban academic medical center.

Hysterectomy rates also vary from country to country. Even just comparing Western countries, all with relatively sophisticated medical systems, rates are six times higher in some nations than in others. The highest rates are in the United States and the lowest in Norway, Sweden, and England. In the United States, the total rate for hysterectomy is higher for African American women than for whites. This may be related to genetic factors; for example, a greater percentage of African American women than white women have uterine fibroids.

RECENT TRENDS

A focus on the cost of health care has led to enormous changes in the culture of medicine for health care providers and patients alike. Funding organizations—such as insurance companies and HMOs and other managed care organizations—pay much more attention to the bottom line than they once did. And they are extremely selective when asked to authorize coverage for patients whose physicians have recommended hysterectomy.

Most of these changes have had a positive impact with regard to hysterectomy. The push to reduce hospital costs has led to changes in treatment strategies and standardization of postoperative management. This, in turn, results in improved patient outcomes and reductions in lengths of hospital stay. Increased access to outpatient services, when needed, has also shortened the average length of hospital stay without sacrificing quality of care.

Cost-containment efforts alone do not account for the progressive decline in the rate of hysterectomies performed annually over the past two decades. Groups that challenge the large number of questionable or unnecessary hysterectomies have also brought pressures on physicians. As we have already noted, technological advances have made possible new treatment strategies (such as endometrial ablation) for abnormal uterine bleeding. In addition, pharmaceutical companies have developed new drugs (with the promise of more in the future) to treat conditions such as endometriosis and uterine fibroids.

While some hysterectomies may have been carried out for sterilization purposes before the 1970s, the ease of outpatient tubal sterilization today and the effectiveness of currently available contraceptive alternatives also may have contributed to the reduction in the number of hysterectomies. Studies have shown, alternatively, that women who have previously had a tubal sterilization are more likely to undergo a hysterectomy than women whose husbands have had a vasectomy procedure for male sterilization. This is true in part because women who have been sterilized may be more comfortable about turning to a surgical solution such as hysterectomy. In addition, preserving fertility is a significant consideration for many women contemplating hysterectomy, but women who have already been sterilized no longer have this issue to deal with, which may make the decision for hysterectomy easier.

Demographic changes also affect the need for hysterectomy. For example, over the past three decades, the average number of children per American family has declined. Fewer births in a woman's lifetime means less trauma to her pelvic floor from childbirth and less likelihood of a need later in life for surgery to correct uterine prolapse (this condition is discussed in Chapter 5). On the other hand, the aging of the American population and longer life expectancy will probably offset the declining figures to some extent.

Even with all these factors, hysterectomy is a procedure that is here to stay—although perhaps at a lower rate than in previous years—because some conditions simply do not respond to alternative surgical or medical (drug) therapies. Fortunately, surgical innovations and improvements in care during and after surgery continue to make hysterectomy a relatively safe and acceptable option for treatment of these conditions.

THE WHY AND HOW OF HYSTERECTOMY

Hysterectomies are done to correct a number of different problems in the reproductive system. The conditions most commonly treated with hysterectomy are listed below. The figure in parentheses indicates the percentage of all hysterectomies done for each of the following conditions:

- Uterine fibroids (30%)
- Endometriosis (18%)
- Uterine prolapse (16%)
- Cancer (11%)

Hysterectomies are also done to alleviate abnormal uterine bleeding, pelvic pain, and conditions for which a specific diagnosis is not identified or as an add-on procedure when treating urinary incontinence surgically or when removing the ovaries for an indicated reason. Some hysterectomies may not have a single specific diagnosis associated with them, and there may be a combination of diagnoses that, taken together, indicate the need for surgery. In half of all hysterectomies, the ovaries as well as the uterus are removed at the time of the hysterectomy procedure. Removal of the ovaries is called oophorectomy (*oophor* is the prefix used in medical terminology to refer to the ovaries). (Oophorectomy is discussed in Chapter 11.)

Although hysterectomy is relatively safe, all surgical procedures have some risks. According to statistics from the American College of Obstetricians and Gynecologists, 25 to 50 percent of hysterectomy patients will have one or more complications. Most, but not all, of these complications are minor. Death is rare, but each year more than 500 women of the 600,000 who have hysterectomies—fewer than 0.1 percent—die as a result of complications from hysterectomy or because of associated underlying medical conditions at the time of hysterectomy. Usually a death is related to a woman's general health, including such medical conditions as heart disease, diabetes, kidney disease, or cancer.

Nearly two-thirds of hysterectomies are performed through an abdominal incision. The remainder are done vaginally or by using a laparoscope. The physician sometimes uses a laparoscope when performing the vaginal procedure. Through the 1990s the rate of laparoscopic hysterectomies rose to about 10 percent of the total, while the rate of vaginal procedures remained almost steady (fewer than 25%).

Hysterectomies are also classified by degree—simple or radical, total or subtotal, with or without removal of the ovaries—depending on which areas adjacent to the uterus are removed along with the uterus. The nature of the problem being treated primarily determines which of these different surgical approaches to hysterectomy is taken. (Descriptions of the different types of hysterectomy are covered in detail in Part III.)

THE DEBATE

So what is the debate about hysterectomy? We believe strongly—and most gynecologists agree—that when a woman's pelvic organs are compromised by disease or she is suffering from uncontrollable uterine bleeding that does not respond to medications or lesser surgeries, hysterectomy is an essential tool. The central concern of the debate is that hysterectomy is often performed unnecessarily.

Many factors influence the decision to undergo (from a woman's vantage point) or to perform (from a physician's vantage point) a hysterectomy. These include the variables described earlier that account for different rates of hysterectomy—cultural norms, regional practice patterns, availability of other treatment options, and new technologies leading to different surgical or medical options. We welcome a lively discussion of these issues with our patients, and we are glad to have informed patients who want to explore all their treatment options and alternatives.

What is *unacceptable*, in our view, is for women to continue to suffer from pelvic pain, abnormal uterine bleeding, uterine prolapse, or other gynecologic disorders because of the notion that a hysterectomy should not be done under almost any circumstances. Certainly, if other effective and less invasive treatments are available, these can be tried first. When other options fail, however, hysterectomy may be the solution. We are fortunate that surgical techniques and management have improved markedly over the past twenty years, reducing hospital stays, complications, and deaths associated with hysterectomy. In the hands of an experienced professional, a hysterectomy is usually a safe and effective procedure.

Deciding whether *you* need a hysterectomy means taking many different factors into account. We hope this book helps you in your decision and, if you decide to have the surgery, assists you in preparing for and recovering from it.

Part I

ABOUT THE FEMALE REPRODUCTIVE ORGANS

The rhythms of a woman's menstrual cycle and interruptions in this rhythm during pregnancy and menopause alert women to their bodily functions throughout their lives. When your reproductive organs change or malfunction, various tests provide clues to the problem. Imaging tests provide important medical information to your doctors and help you to understand your own anatomy and how your reproductive system functions.

In the following two chapters we review the female anatomy and describe what you can expect from the range of tests that help us monitor the health of the uterus and related organs.

CHAPTER 1

Anatomy of the Uterus

To understand women's health problems and why hysterectomy is sometimes recommended as a treatment, it is helpful to be familiar with the uterus and other structures that make up the female reproductive system. The focus of our attention in this chapter is the uterus, which is located in the pelvic area between the bladder and the rectum (fig. 1.1). The uterus consists of two major parts:

1. The body of the uterus, also called the *fundus* or *corpus*. The uterine corpus is supported by ligaments (short bands of flexible tissue) within the pelvic region of the abdominal cavity. The wall of the uterus is made up of three layers:
   - the *endometrium,* an inner lining rich in blood vessels;
   - the *myometrium,* the middle layer, composed of smooth muscle that contracts during menstruation to help expel the endometrial tissue; and
   - the *serosa,* the outermost part, a thin fibrous layer that connects with the ligaments supporting the uterus.
2. The uterine neck, referred to as the *cervix,* which lies at the bottom of the uterus. The cervix extends into the vagina.

The uterus and the fallopian tubes and ovaries (see later in this chapter) function as a unit to enable pregnancy. But as we discuss in later chapters, they can also malfunction in a variety of different ways, causing the conditions that lead to hysterectomy.

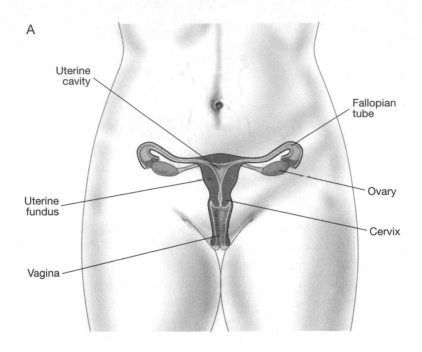

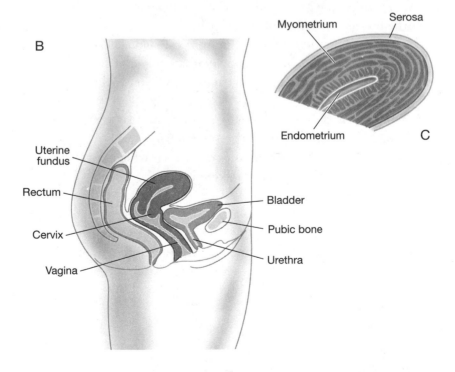

The Healthy Uterus

The size and shape of the uterus vary according to a woman's stage of life and hormonal condition; in the absence of a pregnancy the uterus may range from walnut-sized to pear-sized. In infants and girls before puberty, the length of the cervix exceeds the size of the body of the uterus. As a young woman enters puberty, the corpus begins to enlarge until it is as long as the cervix. During reproductive years, especially in women who have been pregnant, the length of the corpus is greater than the length of the cervix. At its largest, the nonpregnant corpus measures 2½ to 3 inches long; it is 2 to 2½ inches wide, narrowing to 1 to 1½ inches wide at its junction with the cervix. Following menopause, the size and shape of the uterus return to what they were in the pre-adolescent girl (fig. 1.2). Changes in the shape and size of the uterus through a woman's life span are influenced by the ovarian hormones, which have an effect on virtually all the tissues of the uterus, including its muscle cells and blood vessels.

The endometrium, the innermost lining of the uterus, is especially influenced by ovarian hormones (fig. 1.1C). This part of the uterus is instrumental in nourishing a pregnancy. The endometrium is made up of glandular tissue (*glands* are collections of cells that secrete substances; *epithelium* is a covering layer), a supporting matrix (the *stroma*), and elaborately arranged blood vessels. It is responsive to *estrogen* and *progesterone*, the two hormones produced cyclically by the ovaries.

The muscular composition of the uterus is designed for carrying a fetus to full term. The uterine muscle has the ability to expand and accommodate a growing embryo, which will ultimately develop into a full-term infant weighing seven to eight pounds or more. To carry multiple fetuses (twins, triplets, and maybe even more), the uterus must expand further. The muscular walls of the uterus also function to safeguard the pregnancy. They shield the fetus from trauma, keep it warm, and assist in expelling the baby and the placenta once labor begins and the time has come for birth.

Fig. 1.1. Front (*A*) and side (*B*) views of the female reproductive tract structures, including uterine fundus, cervix, fallopian tubes, ovaries, and vagina. *C.* Magnified view of the uterine fundus in side view shows the three layers of the uterine wall.

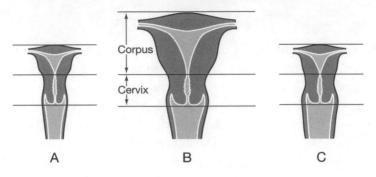

Corpus

Cervix

A   B   C

Fig. 1.2. The size and shape of the uterus at three stages of life. *A*. Childhood (prepuberty). *B*. Reproductive years. *C*. After menopause.

The Functional Anatomy of the Uterus

When a woman is pregnant, the blood vessels that supply the uterus deliver vital nutrients and oxygen to the developing fetus. The vessels that drain the uterus remove carbon dioxide and waste products from the embryo. Most of the blood supply comes from the *uterine arteries*, a pair of vessels that branch off from the *iliac arteries*, the major vessels that supply blood to the legs. As they approach the uterus, the two uterine arteries sprout right-angled branches called the *radial arteries*. Blood also is supplied to the uterus from the arteries that supply blood to the ovaries. Some of the small branches of the ovarian arteries also supply blood to the fallopian tubes, the tubes that connect the ovaries to the uterus. As noted above, the uterus is supported by ligaments (short bands of flexible tissue) within the pelvis (fig. 1.3).

The interior of the uterus functions as a container called the *uterine cavity* or *endometrial cavity*. Each month the innermost lining of this space prepares to accommodate the *products of a pregnancy* should conception occur. These "products" include the embryo or fetus, the placenta, the umbilical cord, the fetal membranes (amnion and chorion), and the amniotic fluid (fig. 1.4).

At its lower end, the inner cavity of the uterus joins with the cervix. The *cervical canal*, an extension of this cavity, empties into the vagina. At its upper end, the uterine cavity is connected to the fallopian tubes, also called oviducts or uterine tubes. These tubes are the passageway for sperm to meet the eggs, and they convey fertilized eggs into the uterine cavity for implantation within the endometrium. The uterus, tubes, and

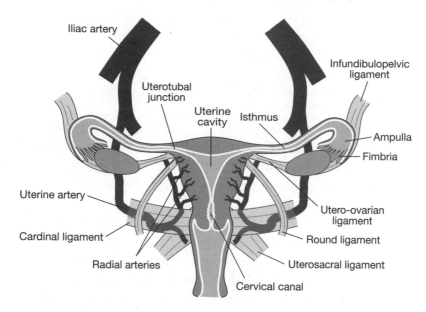

FIG. 1.3. Blood vessels supplying the uterus and fallopian tubes, and muscles and ligaments supporting the uterus and fallopian tubes.

ovaries are contained within a thin covering tissue called the *peritoneum*, a very fine membrane that holds the organs in place like a piece of strong plastic wrap. The blood vessels and nerves that supply the reproductive organs pass between the layers of the peritoneum.

An abundance of muscle tissue also extends between these separate organs. This muscular tissue, which is capable of contracting, is concentrated in three paired ligaments—the *utero-ovarian ligament,* the *round ligament,* and the *infundibulopelvic ligament* (fig. 1.3). These ligaments help to keep the ovaries and uterus near each other, bringing together the outer end of the fallopian tube and the ovary and providing a rotational motion to the ovary. This allows the tube to come in contact with the surface of the ovary, which maximizes the likelihood that an egg released from the ovary at the time of ovulation will enter the fallopian tube.

The fallopian tubes are extensions of the uterus. *Salpinx* is the medical term for these tubes. They are composed of smooth muscle, and they surround a cavity lined by a layer of functioning cells: in the uterus, these cells make up the endometrium; in the tubes, the *endosalpinx*. Each fallopian tube has three major components (see figs. 1.1A and 1.3):

1. The outer open portion, called the *fimbria,* which is fingerlike or fringed (the medical term for this is *fimbriated*)
2. The widened portion, called the *ampulla,* which is adjacent to the fimbria
3. The narrow portion adjacent to the uterus, called the *isthmus*

The isthmus connects to the uterus through a passageway called the *uterotubal junction.* Each of these regions has a specific role in the process of fertilization and reproduction. Sperm cells enter the tubal isthmus from the uterus after passing through the uterotubal junction. After ovulation, the egg released from the ovarian follicle enters the fimbriated ends, which are free to come in contact with the surfaces of the ovaries. The egg becomes fertilized in the ampullary region. The fertilized egg divides (*cleaves*) as it begins its earliest embryonic development within the tube. The embryo is then transported into the uterine cavity, arriving at a time when the endometrium has become hormonally prepared for its implantation.

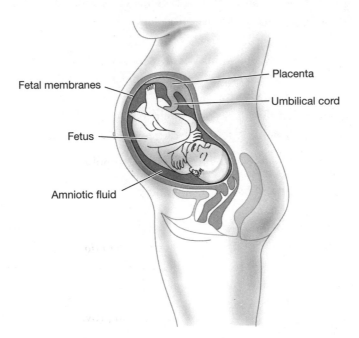

FIG. 1.4. The uterus during pregnancy, containing the fetus, the placenta and fetal membranes, and amniotic fluid.

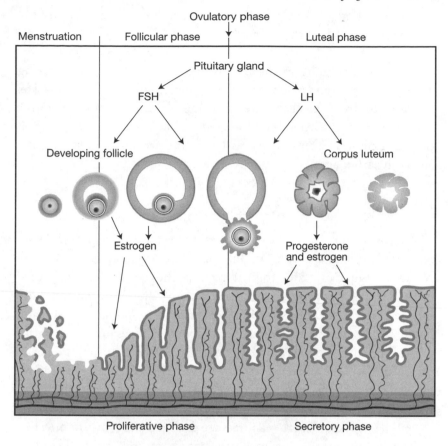

Fɪɢ. 1.5. Changes in the endometrium over the course of a monthly menstrual cycle, from menstruation to follicle development, ovulation, and the luteal phase.

Additional muscle and fibrous tissue support the reproductive organs in the pelvis. Two sets of paired ligaments are particularly important to keep the uterus from dropping into the vagina (a condition known as *uterine prolapse*). You can visualize these two supporting ligaments as a pair of suspenders, taut but with some elasticity (see fig. 1.3). They are

- the *uterosacral ligaments*, which extend from the area behind the uterus to where the cervix meets the uterus, and
- the *cardinal ligaments*, which are composed of fibrous and muscu-

lar tissue and extend laterally away from the cervix and toward the bony sidewalls of the pelvis.

These two sets of ligaments are susceptible to stretching and tearing during childbirth and may lose their resilience later in a woman's life. Prolapse, or droppage of the uterus, is most frequently a problem for women who have delivered children and are older than 50, the age when tissues begin to weaken. Occasionally uterine prolapse becomes apparent at an earlier age.

THE MENSTRUAL CYCLE

A woman's menstrual cycle includes three consecutive phases: *follicular, ovulatory*, and *luteal*. The follicle is the group of cells that surrounds an egg. During the follicular phase, the hypothalamus (located in the lower portion of the brain) stimulates the release of two hormones from the pituitary gland: *follicle stimulating hormone* (FSH) and *luteinizing hormone* (LH). These two protein hormones drive the ovaries to function. In the ovary, each egg develops within a cluster of ovarian cells. This cluster is called the *ovarian follicle*. The follicular cells produce ovarian steroid hormones—estrogen and progesterone. FSH stimulates the follicular cells to grow and replicate (multiply) as well as to develop the mechanism required to manufacture estrogen and progesterone. LH, in turn, stimulates the cells to synthesize, store, and secrete these two steroid hormones. During the ovulatory phase the ovarian follicle ruptures and releases the ovum, or egg, into the fallopian tube. Following ovulation the luteal phase occurs, and the burst follicle is converted into a structure called the *corpus luteum.* (See fig. 1.5.)

In the first half of each menstrual cycle, the predominant hormone produced by the ovary is *estradiol,* a very potent form of estrogen released by an ovarian follicle. Estrogens are delivered to the endometrial lining through the uterine arteries. The endometrium responds to estrogens with significant growth and expansion. The time of the menstrual cycle preceding ovulation is known as the *proliferative phase.* This term is used interchangeably with *follicular phase.*

As the follicle containing the egg grows, its cells produce increasing amounts of estrogens. These hormones cause the endometrium to grow in height from 1 mm early in the proliferative phase to 3 to 5 mm at the time of ovulation. During the proliferative phase of the cycle, the glandular structures become more prominent, and the supporting tissue (the stroma) begins to accumulate fluid as the tissue receives increasing blood flow.

Following ovulation, the follicle, which had been producing estrogens in the early phase of the cycle, shrinks and begins to accumulate fat cells. It is now called the *corpus luteum—luteum* is Latin for yellow, the color of the fat cells, thus "yellow body." The newly formed corpus luteum produces *progesterone*, a hormone very different from estrogen. Progesterone has the specific function of preparing the endometrial lining for the possible implantation of an embryo to initiate a pregnancy during the postovulatory or luteal phase of a woman's cycle. The name of this hormone describes this function: *pro* means "for," *gesterone* means "gestation" or "pregnancy."

When tiny fragments of endometrium are examined under a microscope, characteristic changes that show very clearly whether the endometrium has been stimulated by estrogens or by a combination of estrogens and progesterone can be seen. Not only can tissue examination under a microscope detect the phase of the cycle, but it can also estimate the extent to which the endometrium has been stimulated by progesterone.

MENSTRUATION

When a woman does not become pregnant, the endometrial lining breaks down and uterine bleeding occurs. The menstrual period that results is followed by a brand new cycle, beginning with rebuilding of the endometrial lining. These endometrial changes, so significant in the functioning of the uterus, are governed by the blood vessels that deliver estrogen and progesterone to this layer of the uterus.

Within the muscle tissue of the uterine wall, the radial arteries branch into straight arteries and ultimately into smaller coiled arteries. These coiled or spiral arteries pass through the inner portion of the uterine muscle and enter the endometrium, where they travel in a spiral pattern through the entire thickness of this layer. Estrogen and progesterone influence the spiral arteries. The arteries grow rapidly in response to estrogen stimulation during the proliferative phase of the cycle and begin to coil following ovulation, since the vessels elongate at a faster rate than the endometrium grows. Twenty-four hours before menstruation these spiral arteries constrict. The constriction of the arteries results in a decrease in the amount of oxygen and nutrients delivered to the endometrium. Without sufficient oxygen and nutrients, the endometrium ultimately degenerates, and menstruation occurs.

With today's sophisticated imaging tools, the various phases of the menstrual cycle can be accurately visualized and examined, and therefore we know more about a woman's reproductive system than ever before. In the next chapter we explain how these tools are used to diagnose problems in the uterus.

MAJOR POINTS

- The primary biological function of the uterus is to support a pregnancy.
- Without pregnancy, menstruation occurs at the end of each menstrual cycle.
- The uterosacral and cardinal ligaments are attached to the uterus and support it in the abdominal cavity.
- The fallopian tubes are extensions of the uterus and are made of the same type of tissue.
- The cavity of the uterus joins the interior surface of the tubes at the top and with the canal of the cervix at its lower end.

CHAPTER 2

Looking at the Uterus

Imaging and Diagnosis

Modern medical science has given us not only treatments and cures for many diseases but also a dazzling array of diagnostic tools that help detect problems in their earliest stages and point the way to the most effective and least invasive treatments possible. Some of these tests are simple and straightforward; others are more technically complicated. We believe it is important for women to be able to learn as much as they want to know about each procedure, in order to prepare, to have reasonable expectations, and to avoid unexpected surprises.

In this chapter we explain the examinations and tests that are used to identify problems in the uterus and surrounding areas. We tell you what each test is designed to show, what preparation (if any) is needed, how and where the test is done, what you may experience, any possible complications, and what you should do if there are any problems after the test. In each of the chapters in Part II, we indicate which of these tests may be performed to diagnose the specific disorders described in these chapters. As you read about the different conditions, you may wish to refer to this chapter for more information about any of these procedures.

We start with the most common gynecologic diagnostic tool—visual and manual examination of the vagina and cervix. Then we review other ways to visualize the uterus and explain more general imaging techniques that can be used, such as CT scanning and MRI. Finally, we detail some of the more invasive specialized gynecologic procedures used in diagnosis. Most physicians recommend beginning with the least invasive test and moving to more invasive tests as necessary, but some problems call for a less gradual approach. More than one test may be needed to understand the symptoms that are occurring and to identify the problem more fully.

Whenever you are scheduled to have a test, it is a good idea to review information about the test with your doctor ahead of time. Your doctor may give you some tips for being comfortable and obtaining the best results, based on his experience with these tests. Find out who will review the results, when your doctor will be notified, and how and when you'll find out the results of the test and what the results mean.

A note to begin: After any general anesthesia, you shouldn't drive for at least twenty-four hours.

PELVIC EXAMINATION

The *pelvic examination*, also called an *internal examination*, is a routine part of a woman's gynecologic care. For most women we recommend a pelvic exam every year, as part of an annual checkup; some women need more frequent exams to monitor a specific condition. Usually before the examination you will remove your clothes, put on a gown, and lie on your back on a special examining table that has foot rests (stirrups) on either side at the bottom of the table. Your doctor will cover you with a sheet and ask you to put your feet in the stirrups, slide your hips down to the end of the table, and let your knees fall apart.

This is not exactly the most comfortable and dignified position a woman wants to find herself in, but it allows the health care provider to view the reproductive structures. The examination doesn't take very long and usually isn't painful, but some women dread it. One of the ways to make it easier is to relax, taking slow, deep breaths and consciously relaxing your shoulders, your abdomen, your thigh muscles. Along with the person performing the exam, a nurse or aide is generally in the room with you and may comfort you by holding your hand if you are nervous.

There are three steps to the pelvic exam:

1. Visual exam
2. Speculum exam
3. Bimanual exam

The visual examination of the external genital area is carried out to check for irritation, infection, discharge, cysts, warts, or visible signs of other problems.

The speculum is an instrument made of plastic or metal that looks a bit like a duck's bill. After the visual exam, the examiner will slide the speculum into the vagina and open it; in this position, the speculum separates the walls of the vagina and holds them apart to allow a view of the cervix. Some women dislike this part of the exam, but if you relax, only a minimum of discomfort is involved. A metal speculum can be cold, but your doctor will usually warm it to body temperature for you by rinsing it under warm water. The plastic speculum doesn't go in as easily and may pinch more, but it is disposable and may be used in offices that don't have an autoclave for sterilizing instruments.

By using the speculum, your doctor can see if there is any irritation or abnormal discharge from the cervix. Although comprehensive testing for sexually transmitted diseases may not be the purpose of most pelvic exams, during the speculum examination samples of cervical mucus can be collected on a cotton swab to transfer to a culture medium or slide to be tested for evidence of gonorrhea, human papilloma virus, chlamydia, or other infectious conditions. During this part of the examination a sample of superficial cells is removed from the surface of the cervix for the *Pap test* (explained later in this chapter).

After the doctor removes the speculum, she will do the *bimanual* (meaning *two-handed*) exam, inserting one or two gloved fingers into the vagina and pressing against them with the other hand, which has been placed on the lower abdomen. In a few minutes of palpation, she can feel the size, shape, and position of the uterus and determine if any swelling in the fallopian tubes, ovarian enlargement, or any palpable growths such as cysts or tumors (including fibroids) exist in the reproductive organs. She can also find out if there is any tenderness in this region. As the last part of this portion of the pelvic exam, the doctor may perform a rectovaginal exam, inserting a gloved finger in the rectum to assess the muscles between the vagina and rectum and determine if there are any abnormalities behind the uterus or on the lower wall of the vagina. Although the bimanual exam is not painful, you will feel pressure, and some women find it uncomfortable.

Once the pelvic exam is completed, most doctors will ask a woman to dress and return to an office to discuss the examination findings. Although the pelvic examination is not a definitive diagnostic tool, very often the clinician can detect many abnormalities from a pelvic exam, and these findings will point the way to the need for any further tests.

CERVICAL TESTS
Pap Test

The Pap test, often referred to as the *Pap smear,* is one of the most commonly performed and beneficial screening tests. It is named for George Papanicolaou, the physician who originally devised the test. A sample of cells is taken from the cervix and examined under a microscope to detect any abnormalities, ranging from minor and transient cell changes to cancer of the cervix.

Widespread use of Pap smears has considerably improved our ability to identify cervical cancer and precancerous lesions. Currently cancers are often detected much earlier than they would be without the test, and cancers that are detected early are much easier to cure. The mortality rate from cervical cancer has declined by as much as 70 percent over the past fifty years, primarily as a result of Pap testing.

The Pap smear also identifies precancerous conditions, alerting a woman and her doctor to the need for treatment to prevent cancer. But the test is not infallible, and not all women get it regularly, as recommended. The American College of Obstetricians and Gynecologists (ACOG) and the American Cancer Society (ACS) recommend that women begin getting Pap smears at age 18 or when they become sexually active. We recommend that most women have a Pap smear done annually.

Certain factors have been associated with the development of cervical cancer. If you have one of these risk factors, then frequent (at least yearly) Pap smears are especially important: women who have had multiple sexual partners or whose male sexual partners have had multiple sexual partners; women who began sexual intercourse at an early age; women whose male partners have had other sex partners with cervical cancer; women with prior HPV infection (discussed later in this chapter) or condylomata (viral warts); women with current or prior herpes infection; women infected with HIV virus; women with a history of other sexually transmitted diseases; women whose immune systems are suppressed (for example, those on corticosteroids or chemotherapy, those who have received a renal transplant); smokers or women with

substance abuse problems; and women with a history of cervical dysplasia (see Chapter 8), cervical cancer, or endometrial, vaginal, or vul-
var cancer.

If you are at low risk for cervical cancer and have had three consecutive normal smears, you may reduce the frequency of Pap tests—but not
the frequency of annual exams. It's still important to get an annual
exam, even if you don't need a yearly Pap smear.

The most accurate Pap smears are obtained when the smear is done
within the first two weeks after your period, so it's best to schedule your
examination then, if possible. For about two days before the test you
should avoid douches, vaginal medicines, and spermicidal foams, creams,
or jellies. You should avoid intercourse for twenty-four hours preceding
the test because seminal fluid can affect test results.

How is it done? While the speculum is in place in the vagina, your
doctor or nurse practitioner will use a small brush or plastic spatula to
collect exfoliated (cast-off) cells from the cervix. Cells are constantly
sloughed off the cervix and are regularly replaced by new cells. This
"smear" of cells is transferred to a microscope slide, fixed in place with
a special spray, and stained so that a number of different features will be
apparent when the cells are examined under the microscope. On the microscope slide the cells retain their characteristics, and staining allows
abnormal cells to be distinguished from normal ones. The Pap smear is
a painless procedure, other than the discomfort some women feel from
the speculum.

Since the mid-1990s, a different technique for the Pap test has been
gaining favor. In this variation, the collected cells are deposited into a
vial of preservative fluid rather than directly onto a slide. This method,
called a liquid-based Pap test, has been found to increase accuracy, but it
costs about twice as much as the slide approach (approximately forty
dollars, compared with twenty). Insurers are beginning to cover the cost
of the liquid-based Pap test.

The laboratory that analyzes the cells sends results of the test to your
clinician within a few weeks. Make sure you know your health care
provider's policy: many doctors' offices will send you a notification of
the results, and some will notify you only if there is a result that needs
follow-up. The results, which are determined according to a cell-grading
method called the *Bethesda system* (described in greater detail in Chapter 8, in the section on cervical cancer), are classified either as normal

or as one of several different grades of abnormal, ranging from benign to precancerous to cancerous.

The most common abnormal Pap diagnostic category is *ASCUS*, an acronym for "atypical squamous cells of undetermined significance." This result means that the squamous cells—the surface cells that grow in a constantly changing region of the cervix called the *transformation zone*—don't look exactly right but are not atypical enough to be described as malignant or even premalignant. As many as 3 million women a year are diagnosed with ASCUS, and in most women this condition clears up on its own, and subsequent Pap smears will be normal.

HPV Testing

The human papillomavirus (HPV) is now known to cause cervical cancer, but many women infected with HPV will never get cancer. Therefore, testing for HPV is not a useful alternative for the Pap smear. However, if you get an abnormal finding on your Pap test, your doctor may want to find out if you are infected with HPV and, if so, whether you are infected with a high-risk strain of HPV. Certain subtypes of HPV are more closely associated with the development of cervical cancer; if you have one of these subtypes, you should be watched more closely. HPV status can provide an important clue to the prognosis of a woman with an ASCUS diagnosis. If she is HPV-positive and has an ASCUS result on a Pap smear, she should be followed more intensively with further testing, because cervical cancer is strongly associated with HPV infection and an ASCUS result indicates that something is not right.

The growing awareness of the significance of HPV has led to increasingly sensitive testing for it. No additional procedure is required—cells taken during the Pap test can be used. Many laboratories reflexively screen for HPV if ASCUS is found on the Pap smear. If you have a history of abnormal Pap smears, it would be a good idea to talk to your doctor about being tested for HPV. As noted earlier, certain subtypes of HPV are strongly associated with cervical cancer.

Other Screening Tests of the Cervix

Other screening tests can be used in combination to diagnose conditions of the cervix, but most of these tests are still in investigational phases and are not widely available, except in some large academic medical centers. One of these tests is *cervicography*, which involves taking a photograph of the cervical region; the photograph is then examined under high magnification. It is a painless test and is sensitive to abnormal changes in the cervix. In another type of test (called *colposcopy*), diluted acetic acid (similar to vinegar) is applied to the cervix, and then the cervix is viewed through a special green lens that makes abnormal cells look white, compared with the pink of normal cells (see below). *Fluorescence spectroscopy* uses small, noninvasive probes (for example, a laser light) to survey the surface of the cervix to detect abnormal cells. Finally, antibody-based tests are under investigation to help improve our ability to identify cells taken in a Pap smear.

Colposcopy

When a Pap smear indicates an abnormality, more definitive diagnosis is usually needed. Sometimes this involves only a repeat of the Pap test in six months. But for many women, the next step is a colposcopy. The *colposcope* is a special stereoscopic binocular microscope designed to allow the examiner to view the cervix through a speculum. The cervix is viewed through the colposcope under magnification, and tissue samples are taken for biopsy. In a biopsy, a pathologist examines the stained tissue samples on microscope slides and identifies abnormalities. More sophisticated colposcopes have a video attachment that transmits the picture to a nearby monitor for improved viewing.

How is it done? Colposcopy can be done in a doctor's office and does not require any special preparation or anesthesia. You will lie on the examining table, as for a pelvic exam, and the speculum will be inserted. Then the cervix and adjacent vaginal tissues are rinsed with a dilute solution of acetic acid to remove overlying mucus and to highlight abnormal cells. A light is aimed at the cervix, and the colposcope is put in place so the doctor can look through the eyepiece and see the cervical region. The magnified image allows detection of abnormal cells, which usually appear white after exposure to the acetic acid solution. Samples of these tissues are removed with a biopsy forceps, an instrument that plucks a small fragment of tissue from the suspicious-appearing areas on the surface of the cervix identified during the colposcopy. This process is called a *biopsy*. The *curette*, a thin, scooplike instrument, also removes samples of tissue from the lining of the endocervical canal (a process called *endocervical curettage,* or ECC). The tissue collected from the endocervical canal and from the surface of the cervix is sent to the pathology laboratory for microscopic examination to determine whether it is benign or malignant. Results will be sent to your doctor, who will communicate them to you.

You may see a brownish discharge afterward. This comes from an iron solution that may have been applied to prevent bleeding at the biopsy site. Usually your doctor will advise you to abstain from sexual intercourse, douching, and using tampons for one to two weeks after the procedure to prevent infection.

Endometrial Biopsy

For problems of abnormal bleeding, one of the first diagnostic avenues is an endometrial biopsy. In this procedure, a sample of the lining of the uterus is removed for examination under a microscope by a pathologist.

How is it done? Performed in the office without any need for anesthesia, the procedure is simple. You will lie on an examining table, and the speculum will be inserted. The physician will pass a plastic, flexible strawlike instrument, through the opening of the cervix and then apply a gentle suction to collect tissue for diagnostic purposes. You may feel a slight cramping during the procedure, followed by transient spotting for a few days afterward. Your doctor may prescribe a mild pain reliever for you to take an hour before the biopsy. You will be able to leave the office just a few minutes after the biopsy is completed. Ask your doctor when you can expect to receive the biopsy results and to learn about any additional steps you should take. Avoid sexual intercourse, douching, and tampons for one to two weeks after the procedure. The laboratory report generally reaches the doctor's office within three to five days.

Although endometrial biopsy is almost always a safe procedure, there is a small possibility that the uterus may be injured or perforated by the biopsy instrument or that you may develop an infection or bleeding. Call the doctor immediately if you are bleeding heavily from the uterus or if you develop a fever or are in significant pain.

IMAGING TECHNIQUES

Sonography (Ultrasound and Transvaginal Ultrasound)

Sonography, also called *ultrasonography* or *ultrasound scanning,* uses high-frequency sound waves and the echoes they create when they bounce off body tissue to create a picture of internal organs. Widely used in medicine, sonography is especially effective for visualizing soft tissue that does not show up well on X-rays. It is painless and noninvasive and is performed in the office of your gynecologist or a radiologist who will assess the images. Many women are familiar with ultrasound from seeing the images of their fetuses that are taken via sonography during pregnancy.

How is it done? In evaluating the uterus and adjacent areas, ultrasound can take one of two approaches. In the abdominal method, high-frequency waves pass through the body with the aid of a transducer, a wandlike device moved back and forth on the abdomen. You will lie on your back, and a thin jellylike substance will be applied to the skin on your abdomen to improve the contact between your body and the transducer. This gel may feel a bit cold, but that is the only discomfort involved with this procedure, and it is very minor. (Some ultrasound technicians warm the gel.) When the uterus is the object of the ultrasound, you will be asked to have a full bladder at the time of the procedure, because a full bladder helps produce a clearer image. The transducer is hooked up to a computer, and the monitor displays the image as it is received.

The *transvaginal ultrasound* is a variation in which a condom-covered probe containing the transducer is passed into the vagina and visualizes the uterus from this internal perspective. Some women may experience slight discomfort as the probe is maneuvered into the vagina (you may be asked to do the insertion yourself to decrease your discomfort.) The probe is rinsed with warm water or coated with a gel before it is inserted. Transvaginal ultrasound is particularly useful for measuring the thickness of the endometrium—known as the *endometrial stripe.* This measurement is a consideration in diagnosing endometrial hyperplasia (discussed in Chapter 6) or endometrial cancer because the endometrium often becomes thicker in these disorders. But this test is not definitive for diagnosing these disorders and should be used along with other tests.

Ultrasound is also a valuable tool in detecting fibroid tumors, which show up as a different shade of gray from the rest of the uterus, often with irregular boundaries. The ultrasound technician can take measurements and provide the doctor with numerical dimensions to describe the various findings. Ultrasound is helpful in tracking the growth of fibroids or other conditions in successive sonograms, so that size and shape of fibroids, cysts, tumors, or the entire uterus can be compared over time. Ultrasound also can use sound waves to evaluate movement in organs, such as blood flowing through blood vessels. This process, called *Doppler ultrasound,* is helpful in diagnosing cancer because malignant tumors can be differentiated from benign conditions by the detection of blood vessels with high blood flow located in places where they are not supposed to be located.

Because transvaginal ultrasound is a safe and relatively noninvasive procedure, it is often one of the first tests your doctor will order. Usually an ultrasound procedure takes about fifteen to thirty minutes. After an ultrasound procedure a woman can resume her normal activities.

Computed Axial Tomography (CT Scan)

CT scanning (also commonly known as CAT scanning) is a special X-ray process that generates a three-dimensional image. Like any X-ray, the CT scan is painless and poses little, if any, risk to the person having it. While the person lies on her back, an X-ray tube rotates in a circle around the body, taking multiple pictures as it turns, as if making "slices" at different levels of the body. The pictures are then reconstructed on a computer, where the radiologist interpreting them sees successive slices or cross sections of the part of the body being imaged. CT scans can provide information about the size or shape of the uterus or fibroids or other tumors. CT scanning is valuable in its ability to look at soft tissue, bone, and blood vessels, but it is a relatively expensive procedure. CT scanners are found at most hospitals and at sophisticated imaging centers. Today many centers are even offering total body CT scanning.

How is it done? When you get a CT scan, you lie on a table that is moved slowly into the scanner, which looks like a large hollow cylinder lying upright. Usually you are not required to remove your clothes. Your doctor will tell you of any specific preparation. Often patients are asked not to eat solid food for six hours before a pelvic scan, so the bowel does not move during the imaging. (An active bowel will cause the individual X-ray slices to be out of focus, just like what happens in a photograph when there is movement as the photograph is taken.) An intravenous line may be inserted if contrast dye is going to be injected.

Your scan will be interpreted by a radiologist, who will communicate with your health care provider about the findings.

Magnetic Resonance Imaging (MRI)

MRI produces clear, detailed pictures of the organs and other structures in the body by using a powerful magnetic field, radio waves, and a computer to create cross-sectional images. It is based on the principles of nuclear magnetic resonance, a technique scientists use to gain microscopic information about molecules. It is better than X-rays at imaging soft tissue and is sometimes useful for looking at the uterus and surrounding areas.

No special preparation is needed for an MRI, but you might want to bring a relaxing CD with you. Some centers will provide stereo headphones with music. You will be advised to eat as usual and to wear loose, comfortable clothing without any metal fastenings and no jewelry. No metal is allowed in the proximity of the MRI because it would be attracted to the strong magnet. If you have metal in your body, such as screws or plates from previous surgery, metal fragments from injuries, some dental bridgework, or a pacemaker, you may not be a candidate for MRI.

How is it done? For the procedure you will lie on a table that moves into a tunnel-shaped magnet approximately 24 inches in diameter. Some people have difficulty being confined to this enclosure for the thirty to sixty minutes needed for an MRI: if you have experienced feelings of claustrophobia in small places, you should tell your doctor about it if MRI is recommended. You can ask for a blindfold or bring your own; this helps many people who are uncomfortable in small places. Some centers offer open machines for MRI, but the results may not be as reliable as with conventional equipment.

Within the tunnel, you will hear loud knocking and staccato buzzing and clicking sounds while the MRI is operating. Most people wear earplugs or headphones and listen to music to block the sound of the machine. It is necessary to be very still during the procedure so that the pictures will be crisp and not blurry.

The MRI images will be interpreted by a radiologist, who will communicate the findings to your health care provider.

SPECIALIZED GYNECOLOGIC TESTS

Hysterosalpingogram (HSG)

Hystero means "relating to the uterus"; *salpingo* refers to the fallopian tubes. HSG is an X-ray procedure that uses a contrast dye containing iodine to examine these two structures. It shows whether the tubes are clear and open and is most commonly used to evaluate women who are having trouble conceiving. It can also provide a good image of the uterine cavity (its size and shape) as well as information about the cause of heavy bleeding, painful menstruation, or amenorrhea (no menstrual periods). An enlarged or irregularly shaped cavity usually indicates the presence of fibroids.

Although HSG is primarily a diagnostic procedure, it may also serve a therapeutic purpose for infertile women. Sometimes when the tubes are distended by the pressure of the dye passing through them, this pressure dislodges mucus that has been obstructing the tube. If a woman is unable to conceive because a mucous plug obstructs her tubes, the procedure may flush out the plug and open the tubes, facilitating conception.

Your gynecologist or a radiologist will usually do an HSG procedure within the first week after the conclusion of your menstrual period. Timing the test after your menstrual bleeding stops and before ovulation will yield clearer test results. If you have an allergy to iodine or shellfish, the doctor may also prescribe a corticosteroid medication to take before the procedure to reduce the risk of allergic reaction to the dye. Tell your doctor if you are aware of any allergy you may have to iodine-based dye or shellfish; if you have such an allergy, you may also have an allergic reaction to the iodine dye.

How is it done? The HSG is done on an outpatient basis. Many women find it helpful to take an over-the-counter painkiller (such as ibuprofen or naproxen) shortly before an HSG. You will be instructed to urinate just before the test. Then you will lie on your back, as for a pelvic exam, and the physician will put a speculum in the vagina to see the cervix and clean it with an antiseptic solution. Then he will insert a small tubular instrument (cannula) into the cervix and inject dye (about 5 to 20 milliliters in a water-soluble solution) into the uterus and tubes.

The dye is *radiopaque,* which means that X-rays cannot penetrate it, so any structures filled with the dye will show up clearly on the X-ray. Either a small balloon or a cone-shaped rubber stopper at the end of the tubular instrument will seal the uterine cavity and prevent the dye from flowing back out through the cervix. A grasping instrument (tenaculum) may also be used to stabilize the cervix around the cannula.

As it passes through the uterus, the injected dye is observed by fluoroscope (the X-ray machine), and X-ray images are made at intervals during the exam. As the procedure ends, the cannula, tenaculum, and speculum are removed. The X-ray images can be evaluated immediately and discussed with your doctor, and they will also be retained on file as a record.

The radiation exposure for hysterosalpingography is minimal, and the results are immediately available. The procedure can be a little painful, but most women feel only mild cramping. It is a good idea to arrange to have someone drive you home from the procedure. You may feel nauseated or dizzy for a short time after the test and may have intermittent abdominal or pelvic cramps for a day or two. There may also be some bloody vaginal discharge, generally less than from a menstrual period. Your abdominal cavity may be irritated, causing cramps or a mild fever. To avoid infection it is recommended not to have intercourse, douche, or use a tampon for twenty-four to forty-eight hours after an HSG.

In rare instances, a woman experiences an allergic reaction to the dye. Symptoms include swelling, hives, nausea, fainting, or shortness of breath. These symptoms tend to occur immediately; however, if any of these symptoms develop later, notify your doctor immediately or go to an emergency room.

Since the hysterosalpingogram involves X-rays to the uterus, a pregnant woman must not have this test done, as the X-rays may harm the embryo. The test is usually scheduled shortly after the conclusion of a menstrual period so that pregnancy would be unlikely.

Sonohysterogram (Saline Infusion Sonography, or SHG)

This procedure provides information similar to that provided by hysterosalpingography, but it uses sonography, or sound waves, rather than fluoroscope X-rays, so there is no exposure to radiation. It is a useful test to diagnose reasons for abnormal uterine bleeding, irregular periods, and infertility. For evaluation of the uterine cavity, many doctors are replacing HSG with SHG because it involves less cramping and no radiation.

How is it done? Your doctor may advise you to take an over-the-counter pain reliever such as ibuprofen or naproxen before you have sonohysterography. The procedure is done in your doctor's office. You will lie on your back, as for a pelvic exam, and the physician will put a speculum in place and then will insert a catheter into the cervix. She will then inject sterile saline (salt water) into the uterine cavity through the cervix and then perform a transvaginal ultrasound (discussed earlier in this chapter). This procedure allows the physician to see the outline of the uterine cavity, including any irregularities produced by polyps or fibroids.

No special preparation is needed, and it is not necessary to have a full bladder for the test. Avoid eating shortly before the test, because your bowel gas may obscure the images obtained with ultrasound. For the patient, the initial steps of sonohysterography are identical to HSG (see above). The gynecologist injects saline, not radiopaque dye, through the cervix into the uterus and uses ultrasound rather than X-rays to produce images on a screen. Photographs can be taken of these images. The SHG is not the best test for determining whether the tubes are open, but it is a more precise test than the HSG for evaluating the uterine cavity.

Most women experience only mild cramping, though for some women the pain is more severe. Intercourse, tampons, and douching should be avoided for the first twenty-four to forty-eight hours after the procedure.

If irregularities in the uterus are seen in the sonohysterogram, your doctor will recommend further evaluation with another procedure, called hysteroscopy.

Hysteroscopy

Hysteroscopy is a procedure that is done for diagnostic reasons as well as for therapeutic purposes, to treat a disorder such as submucous fibroids or polyps. Some of the conditions described in Part II may be treated with hysteroscopy rather than hysterectomy.

In hysteroscopy, the gynecologist views the uterine cavity through a lighted telescope—a hysteroscope—that has been designed for this purpose. Through the hysteroscope, the doctor can examine the uterine cavity, identify any areas that appear abnormal, and biopsy these areas.

How is it done? Hysteroscopy is usually done on an outpatient basis and can be performed in an office or in an outpatient operating room. The hysteroscope is slightly larger than the instruments used for the hysterographic procedures described earlier, and the opening of the cervix must be dilated (widened) for the hysteroscope to pass into the uterine cavity. Because dilatation is painful for most women, the hysteroscopy is performed with some form of anesthesia (see below).

Once the cervix is dilated, the doctor will guide the hysteroscope through the cervix into the uterus and then inflate the uterus with fluid or gas. This allows a better view of the interior of the uterus. Then the doctor will examine the uterus, looking for growths or abnormalities, and may take a sample of tissue for tests and take photographs through the hysteroscope.

Your doctor will probably give you a choice between local and general anesthesia. Your decision should be based on both your own personal threshold of pain and what your doctor tells you about what your procedure will involve and how long it will take. If hysteroscopy is done in an office, local anesthesia may be the only form of anesthesia available. Local anesthesia involves injecting an anesthetic agent such as lidocaine into the tissue of the cervix so that it becomes numb. Although local anesthesia alone is adequate for some women, additional sedation with intravenous drugs that diminish the perception of pain may be helpful.

If your pain threshold is low, consider asking your doctor to do the hysteroscopy in an outpatient operating room. In the operating room, anesthesiologists are available to provide additional options for pain management, including conscious intravenous sedation, using a narcotic drug that induces a lower level of awareness but not loss of consciousness. This approach to anesthesia requires frequent monitoring of blood pressure, pulse, and respiratory status. Another option is regional anesthesia, such as an epidural or spinal block, which numbs the pelvic area with anesthetic medication administered through a catheter threaded from an entry point on your back between the vertebrae into the epidural space around the spinal cord. If you would like to be completely asleep, general anesthesia may be an option. This approach may require placement of an endotracheal tube, a tube in the major airway (your windpipe) to deliver oxygen to the lungs.

No special preparation is needed for local or regional anesthesia, which is generally considered safer than general anesthesia. If you are going to have general anesthesia, eat a light meal such as soup or salad the night before the hysteroscopy and don't eat or drink anything after midnight on the morning before the procedure. No tea, no coffee, no water —*nothing*. NPO—*nihil per os* or "nothing by mouth"—instructions are designed to reduce the chances of aspirating stomach contents into the lungs during anesthesia.

Plan ahead for your care and recovery after the procedure, particularly if you are going to have general anesthesia. Make arrangements for someone to drive you home. Allow time for rest and try to find people to help you with your daily activities for a couple of days, especially if you have young children.

Sometimes during hysteroscopy, the cause of the abnormal bleeding, such as a uterine polyp or submucous fibroid, may be identified. Growths such as these may be removed at the time of the hysteroscopy mechanically, with a *polyp forceps*, or with an *electrocautery resectoscope*, a tool that burns away tissue. Rarely, laser is used to remove fibroids within the uterus. Another option of hysteroscopy is to remove or destroy the endometrium during the procedure with cautery or laser. This is called *endometrial ablation*. These approaches are referred to as *operative hysteroscopy*. This operation is often sufficient to treat abnormal uterine bleeding. However, on occasion the bleeding recurs and requires additional treatment.

Any tissue biopsied in the course of the hysteroscopy is sent to the pathologist for evaluation. Ask your doctor when you can expect to learn the results of the laboratory analysis.

If your hysteroscopy was purely diagnostic, you will probably stay at the doctor's office or hospital for a couple of hours. If it was a therapeutic procedure, particularly an endometrial ablation, you may stay in the hospital several hours or overnight. After the procedure, you may feel sleepy or groggy from the anesthetic and may have abdominal cramping. You also may have trouble urinating for a few hours and may notice a watery or bloody vaginal discharge for up to three or four weeks depending on the length and extent of the procedure. Avoid sexual intercourse, douching, and tampon use while bleeding and for seven to ten days after bleeding stops.

Generally, you will know ahead of time whether the procedure will be diagnostic or therapeutic. If a hysteroscopy is done at a doctor's office, it usually will be limited to diagnosis. In a hospital setting there are more options, and the procedure may change from diagnostic to therapeutic, depending on what the doctor finds. Discuss the various possibilities with your physician before the procedure, so you understand what may happen.

Complications from hysteroscopy are infrequent, especially if your doctor is experienced in performing the procedure. Any procedure involving anesthesia, especially general anesthesia, has some risks. With a local or regional, the area may not be sufficiently numbed, and there may be some breakthrough pain. Allergic reactions to anesthetic drugs occur rarely.

Some risks from the procedure itself include perforation of (creation of a hole in) the uterus with the hysteroscope and fluid overload. A woman should be aware that after an endometrial ablation, she can no longer conceive because the burned uterine lining develops scar tissue that no longer has the capacity to foster implantation.

- Perforation is more likely to occur if the uterus is weakened in an area as a result of previous uterine surgery or infection. It is very important for your doctor to be able to recognize if a uterine perforation has occurred in order to prevent additional damage to other pelvic organs. Once a perforation is identified, a laparoscopy (see below) may be performed immediately so that the area of perforation can be viewed directly to see if it is bleeding and so that the other pelvic organs can be inspected to determine if any other injury has occurred. If the uterus is bleeding at the site of perforation, the area can be coagulated or a stitch can be placed through the laparoscope to stop the bleeding. The bowel or bladder may also be injured and need repair. In the rare instances when the bowel or bladder sustains an injury at the time of perforation, another surgeon may be called in to help correct the damage, and a laparotomy (operation opening the abdomen) may be necessary. If a uterine perforation occurs, your doctor will decide whether you need to stay in the hospital overnight or if you still can go home as planned.
- Fluid overload is a potential complication of hysteroscopy. It occurs when the fluid instilled into the uterine cavity gains entry into the bloodstream. This is more likely to occur if the procedure is pro-

longed or the uterus is enlarged. The condition is treated with medications to restore the body's fluid balance. Depending on the extent of the fluid overload and electrolyte imbalance caused, admission into the hospital may be necessary for observation as
medications correct the fluid imbalance.

For the vast majority of women, hysteroscopy is a safe procedure. Call
your doctor or go to an emergency room if after the procedure you
begin to bleed as much as during a menstrual period, develop a fever,
or experience a great deal of pain in your lower abdomen.

Dilatation and Curettage (D&C)

D&C is a minor surgical procedure that involves removal of the contents and inner lining of a woman's uterus. It yields much more tissue
from all surfaces of the uterine cavity than an endometrial biopsy. Often
D&C is done when previously biopsied tissue indicates the possibility
of a malignancy. It is a therapeutic procedure, but it is also a diagnostic
tool, and examination by a pathologist of the tissue that is removed will
give your doctor insight about what is going on in your uterus.

How is it done? A D&C can be performed in a doctor's office, but
more often it is done in a surgical center or operating room. Usually
local or regional anesthesia with intravenous sedation is all that is necessary, and no special preparation is needed. Conscious sedation or a
spinal block can also be used, although this is uncommon. You should
arrange for someone to take you home after a D&C, and you should
allow time for rest after the operation. Try to find someone to help with
your daily activities for at least twenty-four hours after the procedure,
and plan on taking at least a day off from work.

The dilatation portion of D&C involves the passage of a series of
small cylinders of gradually increasing diameter through the cervical
canal into the uterine cavity. Once the cervix has been widened sufficiently for the *curette* to pass through, the doctor will begin the second
half of the procedure. (The curette is a thin, scooplike instrument used
to scrape the lining of the uterus and remove tissue.) The tissue will be
sent to a pathology lab for testing. Ask your doctor when the results will
be available so you can discuss the findings with her.

If there are no complications, you will be able to go home a few hours after the procedure. You will need someone to drive you home. You can expect some bleeding and menstrual-type cramps for the first day or two, and your doctor may suggest a pain reliever. Do not use tampons, douche, or have sexual intercourse until your bleeding stops following a D&C.

The risks of D&C are those of anesthesia and of perforation of the uterus with the curette (both risks are described earlier, under hysteroscopy). There is also a small risk of infection. It is possible that the procedure will not take care of the abnormal bleeding it was intended to treat and that the bleeding may become worse.

After a D&C, call your doctor immediately or go to an emergency room if you notice heavy vaginal bleeding (more than one pad per hour or heavier than your usual menstrual bleeding), if you develop a fever, or if you have severe abdominal pain or pain that persists after taking over-the-counter pain relievers.

Urodynamic Studies

Sometimes it is important to get information about the urinary tract, since problems in the kidneys, ureters, or bladder might be related to what is going on in the reproductive organs. *Intravenous pyelogram* (IVP) is a procedure in which a series of X-rays of the kidneys are taken after an intravenous contrast agent is administered into a vein in your arm. The contrast agent allows the kidneys to be seen clearly on X-ray. Usually, X-rays of the abdomen are taken 1, 2, 3, 5, 10, and 20 minutes after the intravenous injection, while you lie on your back on a metal table (which is likely to be cold). Some people feel a warm sensation and experience a metallic taste from the contrast agent. Rarely, a person has an allergic reaction. In fact, the new agents now in use are less likely to cause allergic reactions than agents used in the past.

The prefix *cysto* refers to the bladder. For *cystoscopy*, a scope is inserted through the urethra (the tube through which urine comes out of the body) to view the bladder. This procedure can be done with a local or general anesthetic. If a general is used, follow the instructions given earlier, in the section on hysteroscopy. Once the cystoscope is in the urethra, sterile water will be passed through the tube to fill the bladder. Then the doctor will look through the cystoscope to examine the bladder and urethra for tumors, inflammation, or other abnormalities. The procedure is done on an outpatient basis, usually in a surgical center; you will be able to go home shortly after it is completed. You may feel a sting when urinating for a day or two and see some blood in your urine. The doctor may prescribe antibiotics for a time to prevent infection. Call your doctor if you develop a fever, if there is a lot of blood in your urine, or if you are unable to urinate.

A *cystometrogram* is a study for evaluating urinary incontinence. During this test the pressure and volume of the bladder are measured as the bladder is filled with fluid (generally sterile water) or gas (usually carbon dioxide gas) through a catheter placed in the urethra. The catheter contains a connection to a computer, which records the pressures in your bladder when it is filled and as you empty it. This test helps to determine the cause of urinary incontinence and indicates whether surgical correction would be useful to treat the problem.

Diagnostic Laparoscopy

Diagnostic laparoscopy is a procedure in which the doctor uses a laparoscope, a thin metal tube with a light and a tiny camera, to look at the organs and tissues in the abdominal area. It is used for diagnostic purposes, to try to find out what is causing pain or other symptoms, and can be useful in detecting pelvic adhesions, endometriosis, and other problems.

You need to prepare for a diagnostic laparoscopy as for other surgery, eating a light meal the night before and no food or drink, not even water, after midnight and the morning of the procedure. It is advisable to find someone to help you with your daily activities for several days after the laparoscopy.

How is it done? The laparoscopy is usually done under general anesthesia in an outpatient hospital setting. The doctor will make a small incision (about half an inch long) in or just below your bellybutton and place a small needle to deliver carbon dioxide gas to inflate the peritoneal cavity, which is where most of your abdominal and pelvic organs are located. The gas creates a space in the peritoneal cavity and helps the doctor see your organs through the laparoscope, which is inserted through the small incision. Through a second small incision (less than half an inch in length) elsewhere on the abdomen, the doctor will insert another instrument to help manipulate the pelvic organs in order to get the clearest possible view of the uterus, tubes, ovaries, and adjacent structures or take samples of any abnormal tissue that is seen through the scope. Occasionally a third incision may be needed. The laparoscope is used to look at the organs and tissues and to guide the other tool. Tissue samples will be sent to a lab for analysis.

Laparoscopy has been hailed as the new wave of surgery, much easier on a woman than more conventional abdominal surgery that utilizes large incisions. And it is true that recovery from laparoscopy is much easier than from surgery that uses an abdominal incision. But you'll still feel some aftereffects. You may go home after recovering for a few hours, but do not plan on driving yourself home. The anesthetic may cause sleepiness or grogginess for a while. You might have some shoulder pain from the gas irritating the diaphragm or feel bloated (also from the gas) or notice a change in bowel habits for a few days. It may be difficult to urinate and (rarely) you might need to have a catheter put in your bladder to drain urine for a few days. You should avoid working out and lifting more than five pounds for about ten days, until the abdominal incisions are healed. Ask your doctor how much you can lift, what other modifications to normal life are necessary, and how long the restrictions should last.

The risks of laparoscopy include the risks of general anesthesia as well as possible damage to organs or blood vessels. There is risk of infection or bleeding and also of a blood clot breaking off and entering the bloodstream. These events occur rarely. Risks are usually higher in people who have other complicating medical conditions such as heart disease or diabetes. Ask your doctor how the specific risks apply to you personally.

After the procedure, call your doctor or go to an emergency room if you develop a fever; if you develop redness, swelling, pain, or drainage from the small abdominal incisions; if you feel chest or abdominal pain or swelling; if you become short of breath or dizzy and faint; or if you experience nausea or vomiting.

THE TESTS AND INSTRUMENTS described in this chapter represent state-of-the-art diagnostic technology and can provide important information to help your doctor understand why you might be having symptoms or experiencing a problem. In Part II, we describe the different conditions diagnosed by these tests.

Part II

WHAT CAN GO WRONG?

One of the marvels of human life is that our bodies function as well as they do. From the cellular level up, countless chemical and biological actions and interactions are occurring every moment of every day. For most people, most of the time, those activities proceed in a way that allows them to function and enjoy good health.

But sometimes things go wrong. A number of different conditions in the uterus can cause discomfort, pain, or bleeding or even adversely affect a woman's general health. In the following chapters we describe these conditions. Keep in mind that the diagnostic tests mentioned in Chapters 3–8 are described in detail in Chapter 2.

CHAPTER 3

Uterine Fibroids

𝕮 Obviously something was not as it should be. Stephanie was focused on her career as a lawyer in Washington, D.C., as she had been for years, but when she reached her early forties, she could no longer ignore her physical symptoms. She had heavier periods than usual and vaginal bleeding between periods. She was severely constipated and felt pressure on her bladder all the time. She assured herself that the intensity of her work was causing physical symptoms, but finally she had to admit that something was going on, and she consulted her primary care doctor. After a physical exam and an evaluation of her symptoms, her internist told her she had fibroids.

Stephanie knew she wanted to see someone who specialized in treating fibroids before she made decisions that would affect the rest of her life. She consulted one of the experts in the field and was not surprised when, after talking to her, examining her, and doing some tests, he recommended hysterectomy. It seemed the commonsense solution to her, but she had read some antihysterectomy literature and was frightened. Still, she trusted her doctor and decided to go ahead with the surgery.

𝕮 The pattern of Rebecca's life was clear to her by the time she was in her thirties—every three or four years she'd have a myomectomy to remove fibroids from her uterus. First she would get a hormone injection to shrink the tumors to make them easier to remove; then she had the surgery. There would be relief for a while from the heavy menstrual bleeding, the distended belly, the pressure and pain. But then the fibroids would grow again. She kept getting myomectomies rather than a hysterectomy because she wanted to become pregnant. But she did not conceive.

After five myomectomies and years of living with chronic and debilitating pain, Rebecca decided to do what her doctor was recommending—have

a hysterectomy. She was forty and had accepted that she was not going to be-
come pregnant, but the decision was still wrenching. Hysterectomy seemed
like a final step, and she hadn't wanted to resort to such a radical solution.
Still, there has to be a better life than this, she told herself, as she decided on
the surgery.

Rebecca's and Stephanie's stories are familiar to many women. *Uterine
fibroid tumors*—simply referred to as *uterine fibroids* but also known as
myomas, leiomyomas, and *fibromyomas*—are the most common tumors
in women and the most common reason for a hysterectomy. Approximately 30 percent of hysterectomies are performed to treat fibroids.

Tumor is the general word used to describe an abnormal swelling or
enlargement of a structure in the body. It can be a collection of blood, a
solid overgrowth of tissue, or a cyst. (A cyst is a fluid-filled growth and
is not necessarily a tumor, but some tumors are cystic.) Some tumors
are malignant, but most are not. Fibroid tumors are seldom malignant.
They are composed of muscle cells and the fibrous tissue associated with
muscle which tends to hold muscle tissue together. Fibroid tumors may
occur in any part of the body that contains muscle cells—for example,
the small bowel. Uterine fibroid tumors, of course, are located in the
uterus.

Many women have uterine fibroids. They are *detected* in at least 20
percent of women over the age of 35, but they are almost certainly more
common than this figure implies, because often they are asymptomatic
and not detected.

Even though fibroids are the reason for many hysterectomies, most
do not require any surgery at all. When treatment of uterine fibroids is
necessary, it may be possible to remove surgically only the tumors
themselves and not the entire uterus. This procedure is known as a *myomectomy.*

Uterine fibroids form within uterine muscle or within the muscle tissue in the walls of the blood vessels of the uterus. A fibroid may occur
singly, as a solitary growth, or it may occur as clusters throughout the
muscles of the uterus, like knots on the trunk of a tree. Fibroids may be
tiny or may become very large, sometimes even filling the entire pelvis
and abdominal cavity.

The cause of fibroids is not known, but advances in genetics are un-
covering clues. Recently scientists have identified a small number of

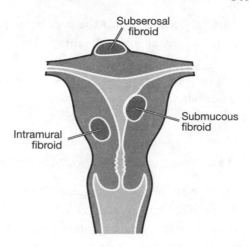

F<small>IG</small>. 3.1. Uterine fibroids in three locations in the uterine wall.

genes that undergo mutation in uterine myomas but not in normal *my-ometrial cells* (uterine muscle cells). Preliminary data indicate that mutations in these genes cause uterine myomas to form.

Estrogen sustains fibroids and stimulates them to grow. Receptors on the surface of the cells in a fibroid bind estrogens that circulate in the blood. These estrogens stimulate growth factors in the tissue of the fibroid and make it possible for the fibroid to grow. This is why fibroids are rarely found before puberty, a time when estrogens aren't produced in significant quantities. This is also why fibroids tend to become smaller and cause fewer problems after menopause, the time when a woman normally stops producing significant quantities of estrogen. The relatively small amounts of estrogen used in hormone replacement therapy after menopause seldom cause fibroids to grow.

How the fibroids behave—meaning how and where they grow—is determined primarily by where they start growing and their pattern of growth. Fibroids can begin growing in any one or more of the following locations (fig. 3.1):

- An *intramural fibroid* grows within the tissue of the uterine wall.
- A *subserosal fibroid* grows under the external surface lining of the uterus.
- A *submucous fibroid* grows from the inner wall of the uterus (the

endometrium) and protrudes into the uterine cavity. Submucous fibroids account for only about 5 percent of all fibroids.

It is not uncommon for a woman to have many fibroids in different locations. The more fibroids a woman has, the greater the chance she will have fibroids in all three locations.

DIAGNOSIS AND EVALUATION

Although doctors who perform hysterectomies frequently see women with problems like Stephanie's and Rebecca's, fibroids often do not cause symptoms and usually do not interfere with a woman's quality of life. For this reason, in many instances they are not detected until a woman's routine gynecologic appointment, when her doctor (or other health care professional) performs a bimanual pelvic exam. During the examination, the doctor may find that the uterus is enlarged or irregular in shape (or both).

The size of the uterus of a woman who has fibroids is usually estimated by comparing it with the size of the uterus of a pregnant woman, using weeks of pregnancy as the unit of measurement, or to the size of a fruit. For example, the uterus might be as large as the uterus of a woman who is six weeks pregnant or the size of a peach, orange, or grapefruit. During the examination, the size and location of fibroids are noted.

Depending on the size and location of the fibroids and whether they are causing symptoms, your doctor may recommend further evaluation or treatment, or only periodic monitoring for size, shape, and symptoms. We keep careful records of the size of fibroids during each office visit to help monitor the growth pattern and rate of growth of the fibroid. How rapidly a fibroid appears to be growing and the size of the fibroid when it is first discovered will determine the frequency of follow-up visits. If the fibroid is growing rapidly or begins to cause symptoms, we might recommend further evaluation or treatment.

Once a fibroid is detected, we often recommend one of several diagnostic tests to confirm an initial diagnosis of fibroids or to obtain more precise information about their location and size. These tests include a transvaginal ultrasound, in which ultrasound images of the pelvis taken through the vagina provide information about the size and shape of fibroids, or a hysterosalpingogram or sonohysterogram. Sometimes the growth is located in the area of the ovaries. If there is any question about whether a specific growth is a fibroid or a more serious tumor, such as an ovarian tumor, magnetic resonance imaging (MRI) or a computerized tomography (CT) scan can be performed to evaluate these possibilities more fully. (All these tests are described in Chapter 2.) The more information your doctor has about the size and location of fibroids, the better equipped he or she is to make appropriate recommendations for your specific clinical situation.

SYMPTOMS

As we've noted, fibroids seldom cause symptoms. When there *are* symptoms, they are usually related to the size and location of the fibroids within the uterus. When a fibroid grows into the cavity of the uterus, a woman generally experiences changes in her menstrual periods, with extremely heavy and prolonged menstrual flow or increased frequency of periods. Heavy or prolonged menstrual bleeding is the most common symptom, but fibroids can also cause bloating, pressure on other structures such as the bladder or bowel, abdominal enlargement, infertility, recurrent pregnancy loss, and pain. Let's take a look at these symptoms, beginning with the bleeding that most often brings women to their doctors and continuing through what is probably the least common symptom—pain.

Abnormal Bleeding

Fibroids that begin growing under the endometrium cause abnormal bleeding for three reasons:

1. They impair the normally rich blood supply to that portion of the uterus.
2. They interfere with the contractions of the uterine muscle.
3. They increase the surface area of the uterine cavity.

Aside from the practical inconvenience it causes, the primary concern about abnormally heavy or prolonged bleeding is the possibility that chronic loss of blood will lead to iron deficiency anemia. (Other causes of abnormally prolonged uterine bleeding include uterine polyps, abnormal stimulation of the lining of the uterus by ovarian hormones, or a complication of pregnancy.)

As we described in the anatomy chapter, normally the endometrium has a rich supply of blood. But when endometrial tissue is located right on top of a fibroid, it is usually not well supplied by blood vessels. As a result, it becomes thin and is often inflamed. A thin and inflamed endometrium may cause abnormally heavy or prolonged menstruation.

Fibroids in the uterine muscle or adjacent to the uterine lining also interfere with the normal contractions of the uterine muscle (myometrium), which lies adjacent to the endometrium. During a menstrual period, the endometrial lining, which developed during the previous month's cycle, is shed. The contractions of the uterine muscle normally help to stop bleeding by compressing the spiral arterioles within the endometrium at the conclusion of each menstrual period. If the uterine muscle tissue contains fibroids, it can't function properly, and bleeding persists longer than a normal menstrual period.

Finally, when large fibroids expand the uterine wall, the uterine cavity increases in size. This increase in size, combined with the irregularity of the surface of the cavity, means there is a larger than normal surface area of the uterine lining, and this, too, may increase the amount of menstrual bleeding at the end of each cycle.

Bloating, Pressure, Abdominal Enlargement

As fibroids increase in size, you may feel your enlarged uterus rising above your pelvic bones, and your clothes may begin to feel tight as your abdomen or waistline expands. The pressure exerted on your internal organs and vessels by the growing fibroids can cause other symptoms as well, depending on where the fibroids are located. For example, fibroids that are growing on the anterior wall of the uterus—the front wall, which is adjacent to the bladder—may cause you to feel bladder pressure, or a feeling that you need to urinate more frequently. Here is a list of symptoms that enlarging fibroids can cause, depending on their location and which internal structure they are compressing:

Adjacent Structure	Symptom
Bladder	Increased frequency of urination
	Pressure in lower abdomen

Ureter	Flank pain (lower back pain, between the bottom of the rib cage and the hip)
Sacrum	Lower back pain
Vagina	Painful intercourse
Rectum	Back pain, constipation

Since fibroids tend to grow slowly, these symptoms do not appear suddenly. Rather, they develop gradually and may become more severe over time. Symptoms can also fluctuate during a woman's menstrual cycle, under the influence of hormones produced by the ovaries, with increased severity from the middle of the cycle to near the time of menses.

Infertility and Recurrent Pregnancy Loss

Fibroids can hinder reproduction in one of two ways: by interfering with the normal transport of sperm, egg, or embryo, so that fertilization or implantation does not occur, or by affecting implantation (the attachment of a pregnancy), causing either miscarriage or preterm labor (and delivery of a premature infant). In addition, if a fibroid distorts the shape of the uterus, the baby may lie in an abnormal position (breech or transverse lie), and the mother will usually need to have a cesarean section in order to ensure safe delivery of the baby.

Sperm transport. Once sperm are deposited in the vagina during intercourse, for pregnancy to occur, the cervix must be accessible to the sperm so they can enter the cervical canal. Fibroids can cause a number of possible impediments that could prevent normal sperm movement. If the position of the cervix is distorted by a large fibroid, particularly one located just above the level of the cervix, sperm may not be able to enter the uterus through the cervical canal. If the sperm *are* able to enter the cervical canal but the uterine cavity itself is enlarged or distorted, the sperm may not be able to reach the tiny openings of the fallopian tubes (the ostia) that pass through the uterine wall to enter the uterine cavity. If an intramural fibroid compresses the portion of the tube that traverses the uterus (the isthmus or the isthmic region), sperm may not be able to ascend into the tube, where fertilization of the egg normally takes place. If the purposeful journey of the sperm cells is interfered with in any of these ways, they may not be able to reach the egg, and pregnancy cannot occur.

Egg transport. Normally the ovary lies adjacent to the outer open-ing of the fallopian tube, called the fimbriated end. Subserosal fibroids, which grow out of one of the side walls of the uterus, may increase the distance between the ovary and the fallopian tube and prevent the egg from passing from the ovary into the fimbriated end of the tube at the time of ovulation. It is also possible for a fibroid to distort the course of the fallopian tube and interfere with normal egg transport in that way.

Embryo passage. Even if the isthmic region is partially blocked, sperm are sometimes able to pass into the tube because they are so small. But the embryo, which is many times larger than the egg or sperm alone, may be unable to pass through the tube into the uterine cavity and implant in the uterine lining. In this situation, the fertilized egg might implant within the tubal lining, resulting in a tubal ectopic pregnancy.

Pain

Fibroids rarely cause pelvic pain. They are much more likely to lead to pressure symptoms (see above list). Still, there are some conditions in which fibroids can cause significant pain, mostly because of interfer-ence with the blood supply to the fibroid.

Pregnancy. If a woman with fibroids becomes pregnant, she can de-velop a condition called *carneous degeneration of a fibroid* (*carneous* means fleshy). In this condition, as the uterus grows during pregnancy and blood is diverted to the growing uterus and developing embryo, the fibroid receives less and less blood and begins to degenerate as its oxy-gen supply is reduced. Carneous degeneration of a fibroid is extremely painful. It can also stimulate premature labor, in which case bed rest, pain-relieving medications, and other aggressive measures must be taken to stop the labor.

Degeneration of fibroids in a nonpregnant woman. Fibroids that grow very rapidly quickly outgrow their blood supply, and then, because of a shortage of oxygen and nutrition, they begin to degenerate. The pain that is caused by this process is not nearly as severe as the pain of carneous degeneration associated with pregnancy. Nevertheless, if con-servative steps (described in the treatment section, below) don't allevi-ate the pain, either a myomectomy (surgery to remove the fibroid) or a hysterectomy might be necessary.

Torsion of the pedicle of a pedunculated fibroid. *Pedicle* is the medical term for a stalk by which a tumor is attached to normal tissue; think of a pedunculated fibroid as being attached to normal tissue by a stem resembling a bungee cord. As some fibroids grow in the submucous or subserous position, they may develop an elongated stalk. The pedicle is attached to the uterine wall, and the fibroid is free to "wander," as if it were attached to the uterus by a leash. This "leash," or stalk, of the fibroid contains the blood vessels that provide oxygen and nutrients to the fibroid. While the fibroid is wandering, the stalk of the fibroid may twist and impair the fibroid's blood supply. When the fibroid's muscle is rapidly deprived of blood and oxygen, an infarction or death of the muscular tissue occurs. This condition is extremely painful and may require prompt surgery to remove the fibroid.

Cervical dilatation by a submucous fibroid. A submucous fibroid on a pedicle can press on the cervix. Then, as it begins to protrude through the cervix, the cervix dilates, causing pain comparable to the pain of labor during childbirth because the cervix contains nerve fibers that stimulate pain perception as the cervix dilates. A fibroid causing cervical dilatation must be removed surgically. Most of the time the fibroid in this location can be removed through the vagina, not requiring an abdominal incision, but sometimes more extensive surgery is needed.

TREATMENT

For many women fibroids require only periodic follow-up at intervals of six months to one year, depending on size. However, any of the following may be indications for more active treatment:

- Rapid growth
- Pain
- Heavy bleeding with or without anemia
- Infertility
- Pressure on adjacent structures

Active treatment may involve surgery, hormone therapy, or a combination of the two. In addition, two new techniques, *uterine artery embolization* and *myolysis*, are now used to treat fibroids; both are discussed below.

Surgery

We started this chapter by telling you that fibroids are the single most common reason for hysterectomy. Yet many fibroids don't need surgery at all, and hysterectomy is not necessary for all fibroids that do require surgery. *Myomectomy* is the conservative procedure in which fibroids can be taken out without removing the uterus. The most important reason for preserving the uterus when treating fibroids is to maintain a woman's ability to bear children. However, even if you are beyond the age of childbearing, you may wish to keep your uterus and choose to have only the fibroids removed.

In a myomectomy, the fibroids are usually removed through an abdominal incision. After the fibroid is surgically excised or cut, the surgeon carefully repairs the wall of the uterus with sutures and closes the abdominal incision. Most women can have successful pregnancies after myomectomy, but in about one out of three women who have a myomectomy, fibroids recur in other uterine locations at some future time. If you are considering a myomectomy, look for an experienced gynecologic surgeon to do the operation. This is a meticulous procedure requiring considerable surgical expertise.

Laparoscopic myomectomy is another surgical approach. In this procedure a lighted telescope (endoscope) and other instruments are passed through small abdominal incisions (less than an inch in length). These instruments are used to cut the fibroids into fragments small enough to be removed through the tiny abdominal incisions. Alternatively, the fragments of the fibroid or fibroids may be removed through a small incision made through the vagina just behind the cervix. Unfortunately, there have been reports of rupture of the uterine wall during pregnancy following laparoscopic myomectomy. This serious complication occurs because the uterine muscle cannot be brought back together as effectively during laparoscopic myomectomy as it can in an open procedure. This procedure requires special skills and judgment. Selecting the right women for treatment with laparoscopy is critical in obtaining success.

When fibroids are removed, sometimes more than one incision is made in the uterine muscle. A pregnant woman who has previously had multiple incisions in the uterine muscle or who has had an extensive myomectomy should have her baby delivered by cesarean section because of the risk of uterine rupture during labor. *Any* woman about to undergo a myomectomy needs to appreciate the remote possibility that the operation may not be technically feasible and a hysterectomy may turn out to be necessary. This happens rarely, but make sure you talk with your surgeon before the operation so that you are prepared for all possible outcomes and complications and you are satisfied that your doctor respects your preferences and will use them for guidance as much as possible.

Hysteroscopy is the best approach for some fibroids, specifically a submucous fibroid within the uterine cavity. A hysteroscope is a tiny lighted telescope that is passed through the cervix into the uterus. No external incisions are needed for this procedure, the operation is done on an outpatient basis, and most women recover rapidly. See Chapter 2 for a complete discussion of hysteroscopy.

These surgical alternatives may be successful to treat your fibroids, but if they are not, or if they do not seem to be suitable, don't rule out hysterectomy. It can be a good solution when fibroids require surgical attention. It is usually a simpler procedure than myomectomy, requiring less time with a smoother recovery. More important, removal of the uterus ensures that fibroids will not recur, eliminating the need for additional treatment, including more surgery.

If you do decide to have a hysterectomy, a uterus containing small fibroids often can be treated by removing the uterus through a vaginal hysterectomy, without the need for a large abdominal incision. When the fibroids are too large to fit through the vagina, an abdominal hysterectomy is necessary. A laparoscopic procedure is one approach to abdominal hysterectomy that also makes a large abdominal incision unnecessary. The usefulness of laparoscopic hysterectomy depends on the location, size, and number of fibroids. The different types of hysterectomy are explained in detail in Chapter 11.

Medical Treatment

Hormonal treatment can shrink fibroids, but it is only a temporary measure. The hormone usually used is a *gonadotropin-releasing hormone* (GnRH) *analog*. This drug is given by injection at either monthly or three-month intervals. It should be given for a total of four to six months at a time, as it creates a menopause-like condition in which the hormonal signals for ovarian hormone production are temporarily interrupted and the ovaries stop producing estrogen. Prolonged use of this medication may lead to bone loss and osteopenia (low bone mass). Sometimes GnRH analogs are prescribed in conjunction with another medication to prevent bone loss.

Deprived of estrogen stimulation, fibroids shrink, only to return to their original size after the medication is stopped. The GnRH analogs are sometimes used in conjunction with surgery as a preliminary step to make myomectomy easier, since they reduce the size of the fibroid. They may also be used in women just prior to menopause in the hope that natural menopause will begin shortly, thus avoiding the problem of regrowth of the fibroids. GnRH analogs are also effective in stopping menstrual periods so that an anemic woman can increase her blood count prior to surgery and provide her own blood for storage before the operation (*autologous blood donation*). Finally, reduction in fibroid size may allow a woman to undergo a vaginal hysterectomy rather than an abdominal hysterectomy. As noted, the recovery from a vaginal hysterectomy is easier than that following an abdominal hysterectomy, the hospital stay is considerably shorter, and there is no abdominal scar.

GnRH analog treatment is safe, but as with any medication, side effects can occur. Many are similar to what women experience at menopause. These include hot flashes, reduced sexual drive, insomnia, headache, muscle aches, nausea and vomiting, memory loss, changes in skin and hair, rapid heartbeat, atrophic vaginitis (inflammation of the vagina related to a lack of estrogen), burning sensations in the vaginal area, vaginal bleeding, bone loss, and weight changes. Occasionally a woman will experience pain when a fibroid degenerates during GnRH analog treatment. Sometimes small doses of estrogens are used along with the GnRH analog. This "add-back therapy" relieves some of the menopause-like symptoms and helps counter bone loss, but the doses should be low enough so that they do not offset the beneficial effects of the treatment.

Uterine Artery Embolization (UAE)

Embolization is a procedure in which arteries are blocked, cutting off the blood supply to a structure. It has become an increasingly useful alternative to both hysterectomy and myomectomy to treat fibroids. Offered only since the mid-1990s, UAE is proving to be very effective for certain types of fibroids. This technique generally is not used for pedunculated or subserosal fibroids, and usually is not advised for women who are interested in future pregnancy because its effects on uterine function and fertility are unknown. However, there have been a few reports of successful pregnancies after UAE.

An *interventional radiologist* (a physician specializing in X-ray and vascular catheterization procedures) performs the procedure. A small angiographic catheter, a thin tube, is inserted through the femoral artery in the thigh and threaded up to the uterine artery. From there it can be directed to arterial branches leading directly to the vessels that feed the fibroid. All these manipulations are done with X-ray guidance to ensure that the catheter is in the right place. Tiny particles of a substance called *polyvinyl alcohol* (PVA) are then injected into the artery, blocking the blood flow and causing the fibroid to shrink. Blood flow to normal tissues is not affected because a network of collateral arteries feeds them. Some researchers have found recurrence of fibroids, but at a lower rate than following myomectomy.

Side effects of this procedure include severe cramping for six to twelve hours after the UAE and longer for some women. Some women experience "postembolization syndrome," a week or so of fever and malaise. This syndrome may occur because of the tissue breakdown of the fibroids and usually resolves within a week. Other reported side effects include infection, premature menopause, unpleasant vaginal odor, damage to other parts of the body from misdirected PVA particles, and sexual dysfunction.

Since UAE is so new (embolization has been used for decades but not to treat fibroids), there are not many studies looking at long-term outcomes. Studies of large numbers of women treated with UAE are gradually being published, but some questions remain unanswered. For example, will UAE interfere with a woman's ability to conceive or carry a pregnancy successfully? Will it interfere with the ovarian blood supply and cause early menopause? In the coming years, as the procedure is performed more often, we will have more answers. Currently, UAE may be categorized as an experimental treatment and may not be covered under your medical insurance plan. If you are contemplating UAE for treatment of fibroids, be certain that your gynecologist is consulted.

Should the decision be made to undergo UAE, your gynecologist needs to be told where and when it will be done and follow up with your care after the procedure.

Myolysis

Myolysis (also called *myomacoagulation*) is another technique sometimes used to treat fibroids. In this laparoscopic procedure, a laser or electric current is applied to the fibroid to coagulate the tumor and its blood supply. Coagulation causes the fibroid to shrink and not return. A similar procedure, cryomyolysis, freezes the fibroid. One study suggested that myolysis combined with endometrial ablation (see Chapter 6) was an effective approach. Recently radiologists have begun to use a new approach to coagulate fibroids using high-intensity focused ultrasound energy. Although still experimental, this technique may have promise in the future.

Myolysis has not been tested extensively and cryomyolysis even less. It appears that these techniques relieve symptoms and shrink fibroids substantially. However, they often result in pelvic adhesions (fibrous bands of tissue that sometimes form when tissue heals by scarring.) (For a more detailed discussion of pelvic adhesions, see Chapter 7.) Some women have had successful pregnancies after myolysis, but there have also been reports of late-term uterine rupture and miscarriage in pregnancies. Any woman contemplating pregnancy after myolysis should be closely followed by a high-risk pregnancy specialist.

MAJOR POINTS

- Fibroids are abnormal growths of the uterine muscle that are generally benign.
- Fibroids are frequently associated with symptoms of pressure, irregular uterine bleeding, abdominal enlargement, or pain.
- Fibroids are the most common reason for hysterectomy.
- Other procedures, such as myomectomy or uterine artery embolization, may be used to treat uterine fibroids.

℘

CHAPTER 4

Endometriosis

℘ *From age 22, Beverly endured painful cramping with her menstrual periods. She knew she would have to spend at least a day each month in bed, and she took prescription painkillers for several days. Each year during her pelvic exam her doctor gave her a prescription for pain medicine and scheduled a return visit in one year's time.*

After several years, Beverly decided to switch doctors. Her new gynecologist suggested doing exploratory surgery to diagnose her problem. At age 30, after laparoscopic surgery revealed endometrial tissue on her uterus, tubes, and ovaries, she was diagnosed with endometriosis. The doctor destroyed much of the overgrown endometrial tissue using a laser through the laparoscope and also had to make a larger abdominal incision to remove her enlarged and overgrown left ovary.

Beverly remembers she "felt pretty rough" after the surgery, and in the next five years she had three more laparoscopic procedures to treat the endometriosis that would not stop recurring. "You're going to need a hysterectomy," her doctor told her, but she was in a quandary, wanting a pregnancy, fearing the hormonal changes hysterectomy would bring. When she was 36, she accepted that she was not going to become pregnant and decided to have a hysterectomy. But she cried as she went through the preoperative preparations and wondered if she was doing the right thing.

℘ *Jessica's two sisters and her mother all had endometriosis, and they'd all had hysterectomies before they were 40. Jessica also had endometriosis and had had multiple surgeries herself, both laparoscopies and laparotomies (in which a large abdominal incision is made). She gave birth to her daughter at age 28, but she had had no luck conceiving again. She desperately wanted another child and sought infertility treatment, but she knew that the in-*

*tractable endometriosis was preventing pregnancy. She decided to have a
hysterectomy, as her doctor had been recommending, after enduring months
of unrelenting pain caused by the spreading endometriosis. She was 41.*

Endometriosis is a condition in which endometrial tissue grows outside the uterus, usually in the pelvic cavity. It occurs most often in
women during their reproductive years and is frequently characterized
by pain—increasingly severe pelvic pain, increased pain with menstruation, or pain with sexual intercourse. It is not a malignant or premalignant condition.

The extent and severity of endometriosis vary greatly from one
woman to another. Some women with endometriosis are entirely
symptom-free, but symptoms generally range from mild to severe. For
some women symptoms are barely noticeable, whereas for others they
interfere substantially with the activities and enjoyment of daily living
and can prevent pregnancy. When the activities of daily living become
burdensome and difficult to accomplish because of severe symptoms of
endometriosis, hysterectomy becomes a reasonable treatment option.
For most women, though, hysterectomy is not necessary to treat endometriosis and its milder symptoms.

Endometriosis is a relatively common disorder. An estimated 10 to 15
percent of reproductive-age women have endometriosis, and as many as
40 percent of infertile women may have the disease. Most women with
symptomatic endometriosis are diagnosed by age 40. Endometriosis is
seen less often after the age of 44, and it is not commonly seen in very
young women: the risk of endometriosis is three times greater in
women between the ages of 45 and 49 than in women aged 15 to 19.
(Beverly was exceptionally young to have developed endometriosis.)

Even though the incidence of endometriosis declines after menopause, it is estimated that approximately 2 to 5 percent of postmenopausal women have endometriosis. There does not appear to be a relationship between age and severity of the disease.

WHAT CAUSES ENDOMETRIOSIS?

We don't fully understand what causes endometriosis. The most plau-
sible theory is that during menstruation some of the menstrual tissue,
instead of being shed through the vagina, backs up through the fallop-

ian tubes and into the abdomen. This process, called *retrograde menstruation*, may be reinforced by genetic factors, as is likely for Jessica, whose two sisters and mother had endometriosis. Or the cause may be immunologic, with the immune system being unable to dispose of endometrial tissue that turns up in abnormal locations. Most often the tissue is found in the ovaries, on the uterosacral ligaments that support the uterus, between the vagina and rectum, and on the outer surface of the uterus.

Once in the abdomen, the tissue implants itself and grows, responding to the hormones of the menstrual cycle as if it were still within the uterus. At the end of each cycle, when the tissue would have been shed through menstruation, it breaks apart and bleeds. The debris remains attached to the tissue to which it has implanted, leading to swelling, inflammation, and eventually the formation of scar tissue. When the tissue implants in the ovaries, cysts containing menstrual debris and blood often form. Because of the darkened brown appearance of the old blood collected in these cysts, they are referred to as "chocolate" cysts (or endometriomas). The sites where the tissue grows sometimes develop into thickened areas called *nodules* or *lesions*. The symptoms of endometriosis include increasingly painful menstrual periods (dysmenorrhea), pain associated with sexual intercourse (dyspareunia), and constant chronic pelvic pain. However, as mentioned, sometimes there are no apparent symptoms—some women with endometriosis are unaware of the problem until they are found to have an ovarian cyst or a large pelvic mass at the time of a gynecologic examination; surgery will ultimately reveal that it is caused by endometriosis. In some women with endometriosis, a nodule behind the uterus, a tender mass in the area of the ovaries (adnexa), or generalized pelvic tenderness is found during a pelvic exam. Often endometriosis is first diagnosed in women when they seek treatment for infertility.

DIAGNOSIS

Noninvasive tests such as transvaginal ultrasound and CA-125, a blood test that checks for the elevation of a particular substance in the blood, are helpful in confirming the suspicion of endometriosis, although elevated CA-125 levels are not specific for endometriosis (see below). Ultrasound is a useful diagnostic tool when an ovarian cyst is found during a pelvic exam or when the exam does not identify a reason to explain pelvic pain. This technology is detailed in Chapter 2. An ultrasound image that appears black is usually a cyst; an image that looks white is solid; and one that is gray is referred to as *echogenic*, as the ultrasound machine transforms into a gray image the echoes that occur when sound waves bounce off a cyst. Ovarian endometriosis may appear as echogenic cysts.

Transvaginal ultrasound can be especially useful in identifying *endometriomas*, the masses of endometrial tissue that form outside the uterus. It may be necessary to repeat the ultrasound procedure at various phases of the menstrual cycle because a normal corpus luteum, which occurs as a result of the ovulation process, can look exactly like an endometriotic cyst on a sonogram. If there is evidence of a persistent echogenic cyst in a series of ultrasounds through more than one menstrual cycle, endometriosis is likely.

The diagnostic blood test looks for an elevated level of a substance in the blood called CA-125. CA-125 is an *antigen* (something the body reacts to by producing antibodies) that becomes elevated when a woman has active endometriosis. The usefulness of this test is limited, however, because CA-125 levels in blood are elevated by other conditions, such as pelvic inflammatory disease and ovarian and endometrial cancer. A blood test that could serve as a specific marker only for endometriosis would be extremely useful in identifying and following the progress of endometriosis both before and after treatment. However, a marker specific only to the diagnosis of endometriosis has not yet been developed.

Thus, although endometriosis may be suspected from a woman's symptoms and history, these noninvasive tests are not conclusive. The only way to establish the diagnosis of endometriosis definitively is for your doctor to take a biopsy of tissue suspected to be endometriosis or to perform a laparoscopy and view the abdomen directly. The laparoscopic examination may reveal endometriosis, or it may be an inconclusive examination. When the diagnosis is inconclusive from visualization, a biopsy of any abnormal-appearing area can confirm the presence of endometriosis or indicate other conditions that are causing the symptoms.

During the laparoscopy, the doctor inspects the pelvic organs and their linings (the peritoneal surfaces) as well as the surfaces of the bladder and bowel through a tiny scope inserted through a small incision in the abdomen. Endometriosis can be identified visually. It may appear as tiny implants (small spots of dark red, violet-blue, or black areas) covering or replacing the normal lining of the pelvic cavity, as large blue-black (chocolate) cysts within the ovaries, or as reddish filmy tissue like plastic wrap covering parts of the pelvic organs or causing the organs to adhere to each other.

Often, in more advanced stages, endometriosis causes scar tissue to form around the pelvic organs, which attaches them to each other. For example, the ovaries might be stuck behind the uterus, or the bowel might be attached to an ovary or the fallopian tube. This scar tissue may result in increasingly severe pelvic pain as the endometriosis progresses and the tissue grows.

TREATMENT OPTIONS

Treatment of endometriosis should almost always be approached gradually, in stages. If you experience pelvic pain or dysmenorrhea and your doctor suspects that endometriosis is the cause, we recommend that your doctor treat your symptoms (for example, with pain medications or hormones) before you undergo laparoscopic confirmation of the diagnosis. The exception to this advice might be for a woman who is trying to become pregnant. Since endometriosis may reduce fertility, if you are trying to conceive, you might want to consider laparoscopy to confirm and treat endometriosis earlier in the evaluation process.

A number of different types of medications can be helpful. These include anti-inflammatory medications called *prostaglandin synthetase inhibitors*. (Prostaglandins are the natural chemicals that cause the uterus and blood vessels to contract.) Hormonal preparations are also prescribed frequently—progestins and oral contraceptives, which can be taken either every day without interruption (to prevent menstruation) or cyclically. For many women, cyclic treatment—taking pills for three weeks, then going medication-free for a fourth week—relieves discomfort and promotes a regular menstrual cycle. Combination oral contraceptives, with lower than usual estrogen content (20 micrograms) and more active progestin, such as levonorgestrel or norethindrone acetate, are the preferred treatment for endometriosis. New progestins are being developed that hold promise for more effective treatment of endometriosis.

If your pain persists when you are taking an oral contraceptive cyclically, you can switch to a continuous daily dose. This may improve symptoms enough to avoid surgery. However, breakthrough bleeding sometimes occurs when the combination pill is taken daily without any interruption, so periodically you may need to take a short (four- to seven-day) break to shed the small amount of lining that has built up over time.

If the symptoms persist, we suggest that it is time to move on to surgery—definitive laparoscopic diagnosis and treatment. Many women, like Beverly and Jessica, suffer for years before taking this step. Often fertility is an important consideration, as it was for both Beverly and Jessica. When this is the case, we recommend that initial laparoscopy be done by someone trained to treat the endometriosis surgically, so that treatment can occur at the same time. This avoids multiple laparoscopic procedures. In addition, it is useful to document the extent of endometriosis with video or photographs taken during the laparoscopy, to provide visual evidence of the extent, location, and appearance of the disorder.

The American Society for Reproductive Medicine has developed a classification system for staging endometriosis (fig. 4.1). This system allows the extent and severity of disease to be categorized through the use of a point system. The subjective nature of assessment limits the effectiveness of this method, but it is the best descriptive tool currently available and is fairly good at differentiating minimal to mild from moderate to severe disease. Mild endometriosis can usually be treated successfully with conservative measures (medication), but moderate to severe disease, which is more likely to include pelvic adhesions or endometriomas larger than 2 cm (or both), more often requires surgical treatment.

Continuing Management

Once a laparoscopy establishes a diagnosis of endometriosis, treatment depends on the symptoms and the severity of your disease. If pelvic pain is your primary symptom and you are not immediately concerned about becoming pregnant, conservative hormonal therapy in conjunction with prostaglandin inhibitors is often enough to suppress symptoms and stop the progression of endometriosis. Hormonal treatment is based on the known patterns of this disease—estrogen stimulates the development and progression of endometriosis, whereas pro-

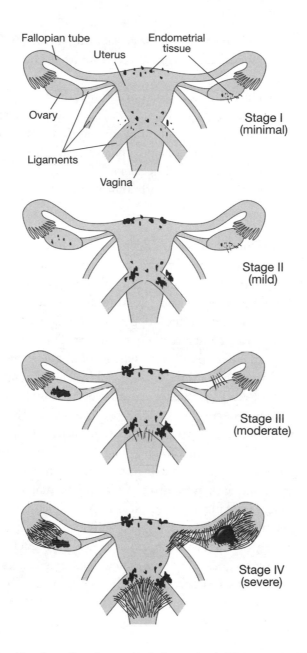

FIG. 4.1. Classification of endometriosis (rear view). The stage is determined by the severity of the endometriosis. Stage I (minimal); Stage II (mild) with peritoneal implants; Stage III (moderate) with peritoneal implants and endometriotic cysts (endometriomas); Stage IV (severe) with extensive peritoneal implants, large endometriomas, and dense adhesions (a chocolate cyst is pictured on the right ovary).

gesterone eases symptoms. Treatment possibilities include the following. If one of these approaches does not succeed, another one can be used.

- Continuous low-dose combined oral contraceptives
- Progestational agents such as medroxyprogesterone acetate, which can be taken through daily pills or by an injection every three months
- Various formulations of gonadotropin-releasing hormone (GnRH) agonists, given in monthly injections
- Danazol, a weak compound with androgenic (male hormone–like) effects

All these hormonal compounds decrease or counteract the estrogen produced in the body and prevent the progression of endometriosis. (As noted in Chapter 3, GnRH agonists may also be used to treat fibroids, but once the treatment is stopped, the fibroids will recur promptly. Endometriosis likewise recurs after stopping GnRH agonists.) Other drug treatments are in various stages of development. These include progesterone receptor modulators (PRMs), which act in a way similar to progesterone, and aromatase inhibitors, which block an enzyme called *aromatase* from converting other naturally occurring hormones into estrogen, thereby reducing available estrogen in the body.

If symptoms persist or worsen despite these medical treatments, it is probably time to think about surgery. The type of surgery depends on your age and whether you wish to bear children in the future. If you do, then surgery should be conservative, restoring normal anatomy to the extent possible, removing abnormal scar tissue and endometriosis, and preserving as much of your ovaries as possible.

Unfortunately, women with endometriosis also frequently have difficulty becoming pregnant, but pregnancy itself often eases the symptoms of endometriosis. If pelvic pain, dysmenorrhea, or dyspareunia progresses despite medical or conservative surgical therapy while a woman is attempting to conceive, hysterectomy with ovarian removal is again the best treatment option for relief of symptoms.

If childbearing is not your concern, however, or if your pain is unrelenting and unresponsive to treatment, or if the endometriosis is so far advanced that conservative surgery is impossible, then hysterectomy is a reasonable therapeutic option. Generally, we recommend total abdominal hysterectomy and bilateral oophorectomy for definitive treatment of endometriosis—removal of the entire uterus, both ovaries, and the fallopian tubes as well as ablation of endometriosis implants elsewhere within the abdomen and pelvis. This approach offers the best outcomes and least likelihood of recurrence. We do not ordinarily advise conserving the ovaries because doing so significantly increases the risk of recurrence of endometriosis. If you are not yet close in age to menopause, however, and one or both ovaries have no visible evidence of endometriosis, the risk that preserving an ovary may cause recurring symptoms is probably outweighed by the beneficial effects of the ovary's production of hormones. Discuss the pros and cons of preserving your ovaries with your doctor.

When the ovaries are removed, we recommend consideration of hormone replacement therapy (see Chapter 13). Even after hysterectomy and oophorectomy for treatment of endometriosis, there is still a slight but real possibility of recurrence of endometriosis and the symptoms that come with it. The use of a progestin for hormone replacement may help prevent recurrence, and for women who have had endometriosis, it is important to use a progestin in addition to estrogen replacement, despite the absence of the uterus. The issues surrounding hormone replacement therapy are discussed in greater detail in Chapter 13.

Major Points

- Endometriosis, a common disorder in women of childbearing age, can cause pain or infertility or both.
- Conclusive diagnosis is made by biopsy of suspected areas of endometriosis or laparoscopic visualization of endometriosis.
- Endometriosis can be treated with pain medication and hormones or with conservative surgery.
- When symptoms are severe, hysterectomy is a viable treatment and a solution to the symptoms caused by endometriosis.

CHAPTER 5

Uterine Prolapse and Related Problems

᪥ *Jennifer had three children. After each birth, she says, her "insides fell out." Her uterus partially collapsed into her vagina, and she wore a pessary (a donut-shaped device) in her vagina to keep her uterus in place. After her pregnancies, her muscles gradually contracted and strengthened, and her uterus went back into place.*

As we saw in Chapter 1, the uterus is supported by the muscle tissue of the pelvis and held in place by ligaments. If this support weakens, a condition called *uterine prolapse* can occur, in which the uterus drops down below its normal position in the pelvis.

About 16 percent of hysterectomies done in the United States are performed to correct uterine prolapse, but there are many treatment options for this problem other than hysterectomy. Other organs in the pelvic region may also move out of position, a condition known generally as a *hernia*. Treatments vary according to each condition, and we explain these below.

For a better understanding of what happens to a woman's body when she experiences uterine prolapse or other hernias, we review some of the anatomy explained in Chapter 1 and give you more detail about how the anatomic structures relate to these support problems.

The layers of muscles that support the floor of the pelvis are called the *levator ani* and *coccygeus* muscles; the tissue attached to them is *fascial* tissue. Another important muscle is the *urogenital diaphragm* (fig. 5.1). The urogenital diaphragm is a sheet of muscle tissue with three openings—one each for the bladder, the rectum, and the uterus to pass

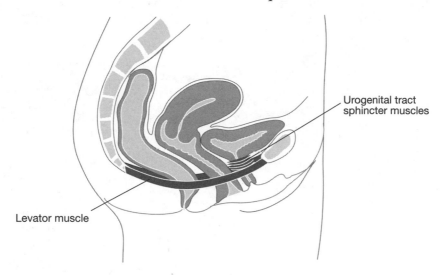

Urogenital tract
sphincter muscles

Levator muscle

Fɪɢ. 5.1. Pelvic floor muscles of the urogenital diaphragm supporting the uterus, rectum, and bladder.

through. The uterus, as we explained in Chapter 1, empties into the vagina. The urinary bladder sits just in front of the vagina and empties its contents through the urethra. The rectum, which is the lower end of the intestinal tract, is located directly behind the vagina. The importance of these three openings in the context of uterine prolapse is that they represent areas of potential weakness, where support problems can develop.

For most women, the muscles of the pelvic floor maintain sufficient tone or strength to keep these openings closed except when they open for their specific purposes, that is, for childbirth, urination, or defecation. However, stretching of the muscular diaphragm and injuries to the levator ani and coccygeus muscles can make the support system vulnerable. Resulting weakness can result in protrusion or herniation of the uterus, bladder, or rectum.

These kinds of disorders can occur alone or in combination (fig. 5.2). Specifically, they are

- rectocele—herniation of the rectum (*cele* is the medical suffix meaning swelling or hernia);
- cystocele—herniation of the bladder;
- enterocele—herniation of the small intestine;

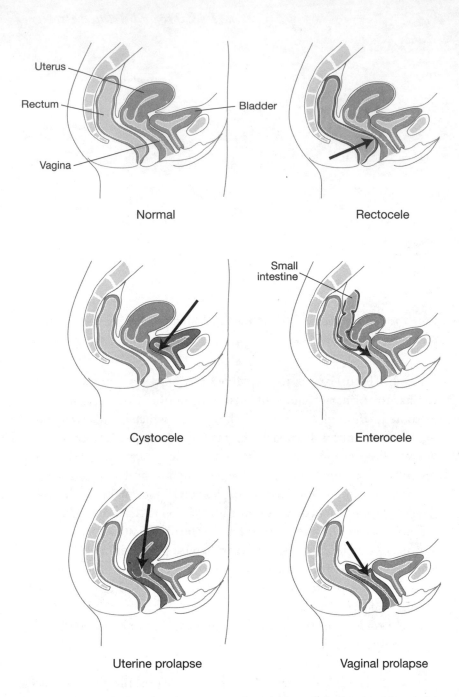

FIG. 5.2. Pelvic floor weakness can cause herniation of the rectum (rectocele), the bladder (cystocele), the small intestine (enterocele), or the uterus (uterine prolapse), or vaginal wall prolapse (following hysterectomy).

- uterine prolapse—herniation of the uterus; and
- vaginal prolapse—herniation of the uppermost portion of the vagina in a woman who has had a hysterectomy.

We define the degree of the problem according to the extent of the herniation or sagging of the specific structure(s). Herniation is referred to either as mild, moderate, or severe or as first, second, or third degree.

Symptoms of uterine prolapse include sensation of a bulge; a sagging sensation in the vaginal area on straining; and loss of urine during episodes of increased pelvic pressure such as coughing, sneezing, exercising, lifting, or any form of straining. Sometimes, when a woman has a rectocele, she will not be able to have a bowel movement without placing pressure with her finger on the back wall of the vagina.

DIAGNOSIS

If your doctor suspects any of these defects, she can diagnose them fairly easily during a pelvic exam. During the examination the doctor will ask a woman to strain as if she were attempting to have a bowel movement or to cough when she has a full bladder in order to detect a cystocele, rectocele, stress incontinence, or prolapse of the uterus. A woman may also be examined while standing upright to determine if she has an enterocele.

To some extent, these disorders are simply part of growing old. All of them are related to increased looseness of tissue, especially connective tissue, a condition that is often a natural part of aging. Estrogen plays a large role in keeping the muscle tissue surrounding the vaginal canal smooth and elastic. Because the reduction in estrogen production after menopause deprives the area of one of its major promoters of growth, elasticity, and blood supply, these conditions often develop after menopause.

Besides aging, a number of different factors cause prolapse of the uterus, rectum, or bladder. These include trauma to the tissue supporting the pelvic floor and surgery on the pelvic floor and its musculature. Another possible cause is prolonged increased intra-abdominal pressure such as straining to have a bowel movement or chronic coughing. Defects in the nerves supplying the musculature or inherited weakness of connective tissue throughout the body may predispose a person to develop a hernia by increasing the pressure in the abdomen. Chronic pulmonary disease and asthma, with their frequent episodes of coughing and wheezing, can aggravate hernias. Chronic constipation requiring straining during defecation may also increase intra-abdominal pressure, as can heavy-duty lifting.

Vaginal relaxation is the term used to refer to the weakness of the muscle, ligaments, and supporting tissue that ordinarily keep the uterus, bladder, rectum, and small intestine from pushing into the vagina. Relaxation of the vaginal opening can be caused by any of the factors just mentioned as well as by obstetric injury related to childbirth. During pregnancy and labor, the nerve that goes to the pelvic muscles, the *pudendal nerve*, can get stretched and damaged. Repeated childbirth or delivery of large infants can make the problem worse, leading to degeneration of the levator ani muscle.

Urinary incontinence is a common problem that can have a number of different causes—for example, urinary tract infection or an anatomic problem such as bladder prolapse or other pelvic support weaknesses. Under some circumstances a hysterectomy is the best treatment for urinary incontinence, but more extensive evaluation is needed before that course is determined. Treatment with drugs that work as muscle relaxants is often helpful. Some urinary incontinence problems may be related to neurological problems such as multiple sclerosis.

Several tests provide essential information about urinary incontinence and what might be causing it:

- *Cystometry* determines whether the bladder can fill to capacity without a rise in bladder pressure. It is done by filling the bladder with fluid through a catheter in the urethra, determining at what volume a woman feels the urge to void, and comparing the volume of the fluid instilled with pressure measured within the bladder itself. A cystometer can measure pressure in the bladder, in the abdominal cavity, and even in the urethra simultaneously. If a woman feels the urge to urinate before the bladder pressure indicates she should, that confirms a problem.
- *Uroflowmetry* electronically measures the speed of urine flow, the volume of urine voided per unit of time (for example, milliliters per second).
- *Urethrocystoscopy* is a direct examination of the interior of the

bladder and urethra with a tiny lighted telescope in order to detect evidence of infection within the bladder lining, defects in the bladder wall and urethra, and lesions in the bladder. This procedure is usually done under light anesthesia.

- *Voiding cystometrography* is an X-ray procedure in which a dye that can be visualized on an X-ray image is placed in the bladder and images are made to demonstrate the angle the urethra makes with the bladder.

If your doctor thinks you need any of these tests, he will probably refer you to a urologist or *urogynecologist,* a gynecologist who specializes in dysfunction of the pelvic floor. By evaluating the data from these tests, the urogynecologist should be able to determine if your urinary tract problem can be treated with medications or if it requires surgical correction.

TREATMENT

There are several different treatment options for problems related to muscle support. Behavioral therapy—in which diet, fluid intake patterns, or voiding habits are modified—is helpful to treat certain forms of urinary incontinence. Biofeedback helps some women recognize the physiologic processes in their bodies and exercise some control over them. Hormonal therapy with estrogen is often helpful, especially for women after menopause, when the tissues in the vagina, bladder, and urethra have become thin and irritated. Kegel exercises, in which you tighten the muscles of the pelvic floor as if trying to interrupt urine flow, often work to strengthen the levator and urogenital tract sphincter muscles by exercising them and increasing their tone.

Use of a pessary is another nonsurgical option for uterine prolapse. A pessary is a mechanical means of muscle support to prevent the tissues in the vagina from spilling out. There are various types, sizes, and shapes of pessaries; each woman is shaped differently, and the pessary has to be tailored to fit the individual. Pessaries may be irritating to the vaginal tissues and should be removed and cleansed on a regular basis. This can be accomplished usually by the woman herself. She should also be seen at two- to three-month intervals by her doctor.

Sometimes, though, behavioral and mechanical interventions are not enough, and significant pelvic floor weakness leads to symptoms that may interfere with your lifestyle. At that point surgery might be the best option to correct your problem.

A variety of surgical procedures can be done to correct these specific problems. Occasionally hysterectomy will be recommended, but hysterectomy by itself will not correct weakness in the pelvic floor; other adjunctive surgical procedures are usually required. In fact, hysterectomy may aggravate the problem unless the defective muscles and fascial tissue are repaired at the same time. Since it is not our intent in this book to review all forms of gynecologic surgery, we list only the surgical options for correction of pelvic relaxation. The urogynecologist can give you more details about what each of these procedures entails and how it can specifically address your problem.

- Anterior colporrhaphy—surgical correction of a cystocele
- Retropubic urethropexy—elevation of the angle between the urethra and bladder
- Sling procedure to provide support for the urethra to increase the resistance to urinary flow
- Posterior colporrhaphy or perineorrhaphy—correction of rectocele
- Sacrospinous ligament colpopexy—correction of vaginal wall prolapse
- Enterocele repair—reinforcement of the vaginal supporting structures to prevent herniation of the small intestine

As we mentioned earlier, most of these procedures can be done without hysterectomy. In many instances, however, because the uterus may increase the pressure on the pelvic floor tissues, hysterectomy performed in conjunction with any of these other surgical options will improve the prognosis and reduce the chance of recurrence. Women who wish to bear children, however, or who do not wish to have a hysterectomy under any circumstances can consider any of these other options as independent procedures without a hysterectomy. There is usually no need for the ovaries to be removed, unless the woman has another problem specifically related to ovarian abnormalities.

Major Points

- Both childbirth and aging can lead to a weakening of the muscles that provide pelvic support.
- Sometimes hysterectomy is the best solution for uterine prolapse, but other pelvic hernias are effectively treated by a variety of surgical procedures designed to address each specific abnormality.

CHAPTER 6

Abnormal Uterine Bleeding

℃ *Teisha suffered for ten years with intense pain and heavy bleeding during her menstrual periods. Her symptoms were so severe that she had to schedule her life around her periods—she knew she had to plan business meetings, vacations, plane flights, long car trips, and other activities for the three weeks of the month when she was not bleeding. Despite her discomfort and the fatigue she developed as she became anemic from the heavy bleeding, she resisted when her doctor suggested a hysterectomy. She did some research and was convinced that she didn't want the surgery. Later she would look back with anger and feel that she'd been confused by what she called the "antihysterectomy hysteria that was out there."*

She consulted several doctors and finally saw a woman gynecologist at a large academic medical center. "Your quality of life is lousy, isn't it?" the doctor asked with such understanding that Teisha knew she would follow her recommendations. "Yeah, it is," Teisha answered. By this time she was ready for the hysterectomy option. "I could kick myself for wasting ten years of my life," she reflected later, and she moved on from a total abdominal hysterectomy without looking back.

Abnormal or dysfunctional bleeding occurs for many reasons and sometimes for no apparent reason. In this chapter we discuss uterine bleeding related to hormonal factors, bleeding from polyps, and bleeding from a condition called endometrial hyperplasia. Bleeding can also accompany other conditions, including fibroids (Chapter 3), adenomyosis (Chapter 7), pelvic infection, especially infection of the endometrium (Chapter 7), and uterine or cervical cancer (Chapter 8).

Bleeding can be merely bothersome, but for some women it is accompanied by anxiety and pain and is life-interrupting. As we detail later in this chapter, a range of treatments can alleviate abnormal bleeding. For some women and some conditions, hysterectomy is the best option.

To understand abnormal bleeding, it is necessary to understand what normal uterine bleeding is and what is normal for a particular woman. There are many individual variations. Normal uterine bleeding—your menstrual period—occurs at regular cyclic intervals from twenty-four to thirty-five days long, lasts two to seven days, and usually requires the use of two to five sanitary pads or tampons a day. Bleeding that deviates from this pattern, either in timing, duration, or intensity, is considered abnormal and should be evaluated by your doctor.

An adolescent girl usually begins having periods before her ovaries begin releasing eggs, the process called *ovulation*. As menstrual function begins, cycles are often irregular in frequency and amount of flow because of fluctuations in ovarian hormone production that result in the growth and shedding of the uterine lining even when ovulation does not occur. This uncoordinated hormone production from the ovaries commonly occurs in many women in adolescence and again in the years leading up to menopause (during perimenopause). Once ovulation starts to occur regularly, the menstrual cycle also becomes more regular. For some women, deviations from this regular pattern occasionally occur after childbirth, when they stop using hormonal medications such as oral contraceptive pills, or during stressful times. However, continuing abnormal patterns or recurrent heavier than usual uterine bleeding requiring use of more than five pads per day should be evaluated by a physician.

At the end of the reproductive years the menstrual cycle becomes more irregular because of *anovulatory episodes*, times in which eggs are not produced or are produced erratically. As you get closer to menopause, your periods are often spaced farther apart, and the flow is lighter. This is the result of decreasing production of estrogen, a hormonal change that accompanies aging. At menopause, menstruation stops and doesn't resume again. Many women have taken hormone replacement therapy (HRT) to control menopausal symptoms or with the hope of preventing long-term adverse consequences of menopause, such as vaginal dryness, hot flashes, insomnia, and osteoporosis. HRT can lead to the reestablishment of uterine bleeding (discussed later in the section on hormonal bleeding).

Abnormal uterine bleeding is inconvenient: it may affect your daily activities, and it may be associated with uterine cramping and pelvic pain. It should not be ignored. It could be a sign of uterine cancer and, if persistent and heavy, can result in anemia, a low red blood cell count. Your physician initially will order tests to try to find out why the bleeding is occurring. Once a diagnosis is established, an appropriate treatment plan tailored to both the underlying problem and your individual needs will be determined.

HORMONE-RELATED BLEEDING

Abnormal uterine bleeding related to hormonal factors is most likely to occur at two times in a woman's life:

- During adolescence, for about a year after menarche (the beginning of menstruation) as the menstrual cycle is initiated
- In the perimenopausal transition, for several years during a woman's forties until menopause

Heavy bleeding can also be associated with other hormonal causes such as hypothyroidism or polycystic ovarian syndrome.

Bleeding also occurs in women who take hormone replacement therapy. Called *withdrawal flow*, it may occur regularly when the hormones are prescribed in a sequential fashion—estrogen for the first twenty-five days of each month and progestin (the synthesized form of the ovarian hormone progesterone) for ten to fourteen days, together with the last doses of estrogen. Both hormones are stopped for five or six days, until the beginning of the next month (five days in a thirty-day month and six days in a thirty-one-day month). This bleeding, which mimics the menstrual cycle and is expected with sequential HRT, is normal and usually occurs shortly after completing the combined progestin-estrogen phase of each cycle. It tends to become lighter over time. However, if bleeding occurs during the time a woman is taking either the estrogen alone or both the estrogen and progestin hormones continuously, it is abnormal and should be evaluated by a physician.

Abnormal flow occurs because of unanticipated hormonal actions on the uterus or because the hormone therapy unmasks a previously undiagnosed underlying anatomic problem of the uterus. When both estrogen and progestin are taken together continuously without interruption, uterine spotting or bleeding can occur initially and is usually confined to the first six months after starting HRT. This bleeding is generally light and irregular. If the bleeding is heavy or continues beyond six months, it should be carefully evaluated to determine the reason for the bleeding and to make sure that it is not related to an abnormal overgrowth of the uterine lining (endometrial hyperplasia; see below).

Diagnosis

To find out whether hormones are responsible for abnormal bleeding, it is necessary to rule out other possible causes such as anatomic conditions (fibroids, polyps, adenomyosis, endometrial cancer), systemic disorders like thyroid disease, or bleeding abnormalities such as von Willebrand's disease, a platelet deficiency, or leukemia. Anticoagulant treatment may also provoke prolonged or heavy bleeding. Blood tests can determine whether any of these conditions exists. To evaluate the cause of abnormal uterine bleeding, we obtain a sample of the endometrium (biopsy) and sonograms of the uterus and uterine cavity to look for abnormalities. A pathologist will study the sample of endometrial tissue. Transvaginal ultrasonography is a technique that has proved extremely useful, especially in monitoring and investigating the gynecologic health of postmenopausal women (see Chapter 2).

Hysteroscopy, a diagnostic surgical procedure, can be used to evaluate the uterine cavity visually and may be done in conjunction with a D&C (see Chapter 2). During a hysteroscopy, a sample of endometrial tissue is obtained by biopsy or curettage. A sample of uterine tissue taken using the hysteroscope may yield more definitive results than simple biopsy because the doctor can see if an area of endometrium appears abnormal and sample it directly, compared with the more random sampling for a biopsy.

Other ways to visualize the uterine cavity, the uterus, and the other pelvic organs include sonography, sonohysterography (saline infusion hysterography), hysterosalpingography, computerized axial tomography, and magnetic resonance imaging. (See Chapter 2 for detailed explanations of these procedures.)

On the ultrasound (viewing) monitor, the uterus appears as a gray, pear-shaped image. It can be viewed lengthwise (along its long axis) or widthwise (transversely). The endometrium is best evaluated in the long axis, the view that shows the "endometrial stripe," which looks like a bright line in the middle of the uterus. In a premenopausal woman, the endometrial stripe varies in width depending on the phase of the menstrual cycle. It is very thin just after the menstrual period and at the beginning of the menstrual cycle, and it starts to increase in width in the week after the menstrual flow has ceased. At midcycle, the endometrium has a trilaminar (three-layered) appearance. It is generally greater than 10 mm wide at midcycle and may become slightly thicker after ovulation. In a premenopausal woman who has abnormal uterine bleeding, a markedly thickened endometrium (greater than 18 mm) may indicate a problem that requires further evaluation. In a postmenopausal woman, the endometrial stripe is generally less than 5 mm wide. In postmenopausal women, unless hormone replacement has recently begun (within the last six months), all abnormal bleeding should be evaluated because the risk of overgrowth of the uterine lining (endometrial hyperplasia) and endometrial cancer increases in older women.

Because transvaginal ultrasonography is a safe and relatively noninvasive procedure, it is often one of the first tests your doctor will order. It provides information about the size of the uterus. It also reveals any rounded or irregular areas of similar echogenicity (the shade of gray), possibly fibroids within the uterine muscle. A pelvic ultrasonographic examination may be enhanced by the use of color Doppler imaging to evaluate blood flow. Malignant tumors can be differentiated from benign conditions by the detection of blood vessels with high blood flow in places where they are not supposed to be.

Sonohysterography uses ultrasound to visualize the uterus and endometrial cavity (see Chapter 2). If a polyp or fibroid in the uterine cavity is the cause of the abnormal bleeding, it may show up on sonohysterography as an area that does not opacify (fill with fluid) when saline is instilled. If such an area is observed, it requires further evaluation by hysteroscopy.

Hysteroscopy, done for diagnostic or therapeutic purposes, allows your gynecologist to view the uterine cavity through a lighted telescope designed for this purpose. By observing the uterine cavity through the hysteroscope, your doctor will be able to identify any areas that appear abnormal and obtain a biopsy of those specific areas. If the endometrial cavity looks normal, we recommend curettage (the "C" in D&C), a thorough scraping of the uterine lining. Biopsied tissue is sent to a pathologist for microscopic evaluation. Sometimes during hysteroscopy, the doctor will see the cause of the abnormal bleeding such as a uterine polyp or submucous fibroid. These can be removed at the time of the hysteroscopy. This procedure is called an operative hysteroscopy (compared with a diagnostic hysteroscopy, which involves just looking and evaluating). Sometimes this operation is sufficient to treat abnormal uterine bleeding. However, for some women the bleeding recurs and requires additional treatment.

Other Treatment Options

Recent advances in technology have produced several new treatments for abnormal uterine bleeding even when no specific reason for the bleeding is identified. These therapies are based on the principle that when the endometrium is destroyed or scarred, it does not regenerate each month, so that the likelihood of abnormal uterine bleeding is reduced substantially.

Endometrial ablation. *Ablation* means removal or destruction of a body tissue. In endometrial ablation, a hysteroscope is used to inspect the interior of the uterus. The endometrium is then burned and destroyed using thermal energy produced by electrocautery or laser. Both of these instruments produce comparable results. Ablation stops uterine bleeding in as many as 80 percent of women treated in this manner. Endometrial ablation is performed vaginally and requires no incision or stitches.

This procedure is done on an outpatient basis in an operating room. General anesthesia or regional (epidural or spinal) anesthesia is given for pain control. Fluid is infused into the uterine cavity in order to open it wider. This separates the walls of the uterus from each other and allows better visualization. A device called a *rollerball* or *rollerbarrel*—a long rod with a ball or barrel tip—is placed through a special hysteroscope (a *resectoscope*) into the endometrial cavity. This rollerball is attached to electrical current, which is turned on as the instrument touches the endometrium. The whole surface of the endometrium is coagulated with electrical current successively in overlapping stripes, like painting a wall. Special care is taken near the top corners of the uterine cavity, since the endometrium is thinner in those areas.

Endometrial ablation is not without potential side effects. These in-

clude perforation of the wall of the uterus by the instrument and injury
to adjacent structures—for example, burns of the bowel can occur with
electrical current or laser energy. In addition, because the uterine lining
is coagulated (and destroyed), scar tissue may develop in the endometrial
cavity and will likely impair the woman's ability to become pregnant.

Thermal balloon ablation. Thermal balloon ablation is a new technique that has some similarity to hysteroscopic endometrial ablation.
Like hysteroscopic ablation, it, too, destroys the endometrium, but
through a different process. Thermal balloon ablation also is performed
vaginally, without the need for an incision or stitches.

In this procedure, a balloon is placed into the uterine cavity. The balloon is then filled with fluid. The fluid is heated sufficiently to coagulate
the endometrium without damaging the rest of the uterine muscle or
other adjacent pelvic structures such as the bladder or bowel. The heat
destroys the endometrium and in this way eliminates uterine bleeding.
This therapy seems to provide results as good as or better than endometrial ablation, with fewer complications. If a hysteroscopy has already been done in the office and did not reveal any visible growths or
lesions, thermal balloon ablation can be performed without the need for
another hysteroscopy.

There are some instances in which we may not be able to perform the
thermal balloon ablation successfully. Sometimes the uterine cavity is
too large or expands easily and does not allow the appropriate pressure
to build up. Before attempting the procedure we will already have
learned through hysteroscopy that the uterine cavity does not contain
any obvious abnormality or we will have removed the detected abnormality. Therefore, if a balloon ablation is not possible, we may decide to
do a dilatation and curettage to remove the lining. Sometimes the D&C
procedure will control the abnormal bleeding.

Polyps

Polyps are growths of tissue that protrude from an underlying structure on a stem or pedicle. They are very common on the skin and in the
colon, bladder, nose, and uterus. Polyps tend to be benign growths, especially when they occur in the uterus or on the cervix. For the most
part polyps cause no symptoms. Often they are diagnosed at the same

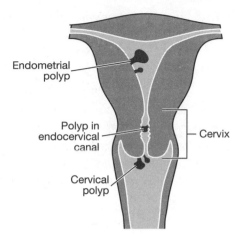

FIG. 6.1. Polyps in the uterus and cervix.

time as other uterine abnormalities are diagnosed—for example, hyperplasia of the endometrium (which is discussed below).

Many malignancies of the endometrium have polyplike areas known as *polypoid projections* protruding from them. Polypoid tissue may look similar to adjacent malignant tissue under the microscope. However, it is very rare for a benign endometrial polyp to become malignant.

Polyps can be diagnosed by transvaginal ultrasound accompanied by the instillation of saline into the uterine cavity through the cervix (sonohysterogram or saline instillation sonography; see Chapter 2). This simple office procedure allows the physician to see the outline of the uterine cavity, including the irregularity produced by the polyp (fig. 6.1).

Polyps are also readily detected by hysteroscopy, which allows us not only to see the polyps but also to remove them. All tissue that is removed is sent to a pathology laboratory for microscopic examination to make sure there is no need for further treatment. Intrauterine polyps can be removed with a tiny forceps inserted along with the hysteroscope or by curettage (scraping of the uterine cavity). It is not unusual for polyps to recur after removal.

When a uterine polyp does cause symptoms, the most common one is abnormal bleeding or spotting in the middle of the menstrual cycle. Polyps within the uterus may also prevent pregnancy or interfere with normal implantation of an embryo and cause miscarriage. These problems are more likely with large polyps or when there are several polyps in the uterus.

🐚 *When she was 32, Rebecca began to notice spotting in the middle of her cycle. She did not have any cramping or menstrual-like symptoms, but there was enough bleeding that she needed to use a sanitary pad. Her menstrual flow began about one week after the spotting stopped and was not different from her usual periods. After three consecutive cycles with spotting between her periods, she had a routine gynecologic examination. Her doctor did not find any abnormalities. Rebecca was concerned, though, because she wanted to become pregnant in the near future.*

Her gynecologist recommended trying to control the spotting with oral contraceptive pills, which usually regulate menstrual cycles. But the spotting persisted, even though Rebecca used the oral contraceptives correctly over the next two cycles. As a next step to find out what was causing the bleeding, Rebecca had an outpatient hysteroscopy, during which several small polyps (less than ¼ inch in length) were detected. The polyps were removed with a specialized "polyps forceps" and curettage to free them from the uterine wall. She experienced no further spotting following the procedure. Within one year, she conceived a planned pregnancy, which proceeded to a normal term delivery.

Rebecca's situation illustrates how endometrial polyps may lead to consistent spotting between periods from one cycle to another. Typically, birth control pills do not eliminate spotting associated with polyps. Once polyps have been removed, bleeding between periods should stop, and pregnancy is possible. Furthermore, pregnancy in the absence of a polyp should progress normally.

The usual treatment of endometrial polyps is removal by hysteroscopy or curettage or both. If a polyp is very large or prolapses through the cervix, suturing (stitches) or coagulation of the stalk may be necessary after the polyp is removed. Polyps alone are rarely a reason to have a hysterectomy. If your gynecologist recommends a hysterectomy for benign polyps, it would be wise to consider seeking a second opinion.

A special situation exists in women who take the drug tamoxifen. Women who have been treated for estrogen-responsive breast cancer often take tamoxifen to reduce the chances of breast cancer recurrence.

Breast cancer survivors (as well as women at high risk for breast cancer) usually take the drug daily for five years after their cancer treatment (consisting of surgery, chemotherapy, and/or radiation). In a small percentage of women, tamoxifen leads to stimulation of the uterine lining, which in turn often leads to the development of endometrial polyps. These polyps need to be removed and the remaining endometrial tissue biopsied, since tamoxifen, despite its preventive effects on breast cancer, has been linked to an increased risk of uterine (endometrial) cancer.

Polyps can also occur in the cervix or in the endocervical canal. Cervical polyps are readily visible at the time of a pelvic examination when a Pap smear is taken. Cervical polyps are common and almost always benign and may cause spotty bleeding, especially after intercourse. The fragile tissue at the tip of the cervix where the polyp is attached responds to the minimal trauma of intercourse with irritation of its surface and spotting.

Andrea, 41 years old, had a routine GYN examination and annual Pap smear. When the speculum was in place and the cervix visualized, the doctor could see a 5-mm fragment of tissue on a stalk protruding from the cervix. When Andrea was asked about possible symptoms, she told her gynecologist that lately she had been experiencing a small amount of spotting after intercourse. This usually only happened just before her period was due.

The polyp was easily removed at the time of the exam by grasping it with a small forceps and twisting it until the stalk was broken and the polyp could be lifted off the cervix. The procedure was painless and resulted in no bleeding. The report from the pathology department was "benign endocervical polyp," and Andrea's Pap smear was normal. She required no further treatment and her cycles returned to normal.

Cervical polyps should be removed for two reasons. Their tendency to grow and cause further bleeding is reason enough, but it is also important to remove and evaluate any abnormal tissue from the cervix to confirm that it is benign. It is common for cervical polyps to recur, and recurring polyps should be removed in the same way. Recurrence, however, is no reason for concern, as cervical polyps are virtually always benign lesions.

ENDOMETRIAL HYPERPLASIA

When she was 52, Anne began having prolonged and irregular vaginal bleeding. She knew she was entering menopause and thought that menopause was responsible for the bleeding. But the symptoms were more severe than she'd expected, so she made an appointment to see her gynecologist. He performed an endometrial biopsy. After receiving the pathologist's report, he told her that she had a condition called endometrial hyperplasia, which means an overgrowth of cells in the endometrium. The treatment he recommended was hysterectomy. Anne was afraid of surgery and dreaded the thought of losing her uterus, even though she was menopausal. She decided to seek a second opinion.

It is not uncommon for women Anne's age to be told that they need a hysterectomy after a diagnosis of endometrial hyperplasia. Sometimes hysterectomy *is* the appropriate treatment for this disorder. But there are more reasons why hysterectomy is often *not* the best choice for treatment of endometrial hyperplasia.

Hyperplasia means an increase in the size of tissue or an organ because of growth in the number of cells contained within it. *Endometrial hyperplasia* is an increase in the number of endometrial cells. For an analogy, think of a village that becomes overpopulated, resulting in overcrowding and expansion of the village. The village would be considered "hyperplastic." In the endometrium the increased number of cells causes thickening of the area. Endometrial hyperplasia is often accompanied by crowding of the cells that make up the endometrium—both its glands and their supporting, or stromal, cells.

Endometrial hyperplasia is almost always the result of prolonged and continuous stimulation of the endometrium by unopposed estrogen (estrogen not counteracted by progesterone or a progestin). As a woman approaches menopause, her cycles often become irregular or prolonged, and she no longer ovulates in every cycle. This exposes the endometrium to continuing estrogen stimulation that is not offset by progesterone, the hormone that counteracts the growth-stimulating effects of estrogen on the endometrium. Anne is the appropriate age for this phenomenon. She is likely not to ovulate or to produce progesterone, and because she has endometrial hyperplasia, she is prone to lengthy cycles with irregular and prolonged bleeding.

Endometrial hyperplasia can also develop in other ways. Women who go through a long stretch of their lives without ovulating but who continue to have menstrual periods (for example, women with a condition called *polycystic ovarian syndrome*) are prime candidates for endometrial hyperplasia. Polycystic ovarian syndrome is a condition in which ovulation fails to occur despite development of follicles in the ovary and production of estrogens by these follicles. In addition, women who receive hormonal therapy with estrogen alone (that is, with no progesterone) are also at risk to develop endometrial hyperplasia.

Types of Endometrial Hyperplasia

Hyperplasia is classified into four distinct types, although the classifications may overlap and can be subjective. Distinctions are made at the time the tissue is examined microscopically by a pathologist (fig. 6.2).

- *Simple* is the least severe category, with an overgrowth of endometrial tissue visible, but the glandular cells are not as crowded together as in other categories.
- *Simple atypical* means the nuclei of the endometrial cells may have minimal abnormalities, but they are definitely not cancerous.
- In the *complex* category, the endometrial glands are more tortuous (twisted) and crowded together.
- The *complex atypical* category is characterized by crowding of glands and significant abnormalities in the appearance of their nuclei.

These classifications range from least to most serious and provide a framework to help understand the implications of endometrial hyperplasia. The classification will identify the severity of the disorder and influence the treatment options. There are two distinctions to understand: between simple and complex endometrial hyperplasia and between typical and atypical hyperplasia. In simple hyperplasia the glands are prominent but are not crowded together. In the complex form, glands are numerous and closely related to each other, a condition that causes thickening of the endometrium. Atypical cells have an abnormal appearance under the microscope; they do not look like normal endometrial cells and exhibit irregularity of the nuclei. The nuclei of cells show evidence of many mitoses (divisions), and the cells are atypical in appearance.

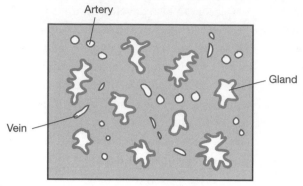

A. Normal endometrium

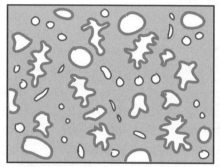

B. Simple hyperplasia

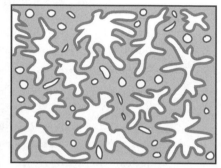

C. Complex hyperplasia

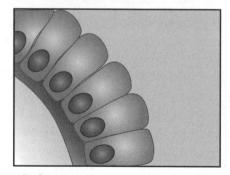

D. Close-up of normal gland cell nuclei

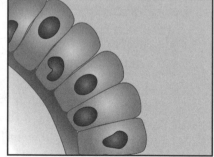

E. Close-up of atypical nuclei

FIG. 6.2. Microscopic appearance of biopsies of normal endometrium (*A*) and endometrium with simple hyperplasia (*B*) and complex hyperplasia (*C*). Simple hyperplasia and complex hyperplasia may have either normal cell nuclei (*D*) or atypical nuclei (*E*). If the nuclei are atypical, the hyperplasia is either simple atypical or complex atypical.

The most important thing to know about endometrial hyperplasia is that, if it is not treated, there is a definite chance that it will develop into endometrial cancer. Atypical hyperplasia is the most likely form of endometrial hyperplasia to become malignant, simple hyperplasia the least likely. As many as three-fourths of cases of complex hyperplasia do *not* become malignant. Even in women with complex atypical endometrial hyperplasia, only one-fourth to one-third develop endometrial cancer. Nonetheless, treatment of endometrial hyperplasia is important to minimize the chance of a malignant change.

Diagnosis

For an accurate and definite diagnosis, a sample of endometrial tissue must be examined under a microscope by a pathologist. As detailed in Chapter 2, a few different diagnostic procedures can be used to assess the endometrium:

- Pelvic ultrasonography
- Endometrial biopsy
- Endometrial curettage, or D&C

Ultrasonography, which can measure the thickness of the endometrium, cannot actually diagnose endometrial hyperplasia or endometrial cancer, but it can help to exclude these conditions. Endometrial thickness, as previously noted, varies according to time of the menstrual cycle or a woman's age. The endometrium is about 2 to 4 mm thick during menstruation, 8 to 10 mm thick just prior to ovulation, and 8 to 14 mm thick following ovulation. In a postmenopausal woman it is usually less than 5 mm thick. If ultrasonography indicates that the endometrium is thicker than normal, especially in a woman with irregular bleeding near the time of menopause, further testing is necessary to identify the cause.

Endometrial biopsy is a simple procedure performed in a doctor's office with no need for anesthesia (see Chapter 2). If the biopsy results indicate a diagnosis of simple hyperplasia, no additional evaluation is needed. If atypical or extensive complex hyperplasia is found, or if a biopsy is negative but bleeding symptoms remain unexplained, further evaluation is needed with a D&C. Uterine curettage is a more thorough procedure and yields much more tissue than biopsy, from all surfaces of the uterine cavity. (For more information about D&C, see Chapter 2.)

The information from these tests, along with a gynecologic examination and information about your menstrual history including whether you are taking hormones, helps to diagnose endometrial hyperplasia. When Anne (in the case described above) consulted another doctor for a second opinion, that doctor had a pathologist who was experienced in gynecologic evaluation review the slides of her endometrial tissue obtained through biopsy. The slides revealed simple hyperplasia or a mild degree of complex hyperplasia, and therefore the second doctor did not recommend a hysterectomy.

Treatment

With the understanding that endometrial hyperplasia is based on persistent prolonged estrogen stimulation without progesterone, it follows that the condition can be reversed by exposing the endometrium to progesterone. The initial treatment we recommend for simple endometrial hyperplasia is a three-month course of a drug with effects similar to progesterone (progestin) such as medroxyprogesterone acetate or megestrol acetate. These drugs are taken orally. A small number of women have difficulty tolerating oral progestin-containing medications and develop side effects such as depression, weight gain, and bloating. In these women, endometrial hyperplasia can be treated by insertion of a progestin-containing intrauterine device (IUD).

After three months of either oral or IUD treatment, the biopsy should be repeated. Chances are that hyperplasia will no longer be found. If endometrial hyperplasia is still present, the use of the progestin may be extended for a second three-month course, after which another biopsy is taken.

If Anne's original biopsy had been interpreted as atypical hyperplasia, we would recommend a full D&C to rule out the possibility of a coexisting cancer. If there turns out to be no malignancy, progestin therapy and rebiopsy in three months, as described above, would be an appropriate course of action. If the hyperplasia persisted after six months of treatment with a progestin, then a hysterectomy would be warranted.

Sometimes hysterectomy is the appropriate treatment for endometrial hyperplasia. Many women with atypical hyperplasia, especially postmenopausal women, may choose hysterectomy, and many physicians would endorse this choice. Hysterectomy may also be the choice of women whose hyperplasia is persistent and seemingly unresponsive to a complete course of treatment with progestins. But it is important to recognize that oral or IUD-containing progestin therapy—treatments short of hysterectomy—are often very effective in treating endometrial hyperplasia.

MAJOR POINTS

- Normal uterine bleeding (menstruation) occurs regularly at intervals from twenty-four to thirty-five days and lasts two to seven days.
- Hysteroscopy is a procedure used to evaluate or treat abnormal hormone-related uterine bleeding. Other treatment approaches include endometrial ablation or thermal balloon ablation.
- Endometrial (uterine) and cervical polyps tend to be benign and are rarely a reason for hysterectomy.
- Endometrial hyperplasia can develop into cancer, especially if atypical cells are present. Still, hysterectomy is not usually the best first treatment of endometrial hyperplasia.
- Hysterectomy is used to treat abnormal uterine bleeding only when other approaches have failed.

Pelvic Pain, Infection, and Adhesions

Today's potent antibiotics can cure almost every pelvic infection, and so hysterectomy is rarely recommended as a treatment and usually only in cases of severe infection. Chronic pelvic pain or pelvic adhesions may sometimes be appropriately treated with hysterectomy. Adenomyosis, a condition that is often very painful, is *best* treated with hysterectomy. This chapter is about these conditions.

Chronic pelvic pain is a symptom, not a disease. To determine the best treatment, we need first to determine the underlying reason for the pain. Pelvic pain is considered chronic when it is experienced as

- lower abdominal pain that is not exclusively related to menstruation, that interferes with a woman's ability to carry out normal daily activities, and that has been present for at least three months; or
- menstrual pain that has been present for at least six months.

Chronic pelvic pain is a very common symptom. In fact, 10 percent of all women who visit a gynecologist do so because of pelvic pain. Persistent or recurring pelvic pain may be caused by a variety of gynecologic conditions, including untreated or incompletely treated pelvic infection, recurrent pelvic infection, endometriosis, adenomyosis, and postoperative pelvic adhesions. In addition, a number of nongynecologic conditions may also cause pelvic pain. Included among these are irritable bowel syndrome and interstitial cystitis.

Diagnosing the cause of pelvic pain may be difficult. It is not unusual for a doctor not to be able to diagnose the cause of the pain from a description of symptoms or from a physical or pelvic examination. In that case, diagnostic laparoscopy is the mainstay of diagnosis for chronic pelvic pain (see Chapter 2). As many as 60 percent of women who have had chronic pelvic pain for more than six months have a normal pelvic exam. Further evaluation with diagnostic laparoscopy can identify the cause of the pain in more than half of these women. Up to 40 percent of all gynecologic laparoscopic procedures are done to evaluate pelvic pain, but, again, even a laparoscopy will fail to identify the reason for the pain in many women.

The most common findings during laparoscopy that diagnose the cause of pelvic pain are pelvic adhesions and endometriosis. Rarely, an unsuspected pelvic infection is the culprit and is also identifiable at the time of laparoscopic evaluation. As noted, for a woman with adhesions or adenomyosis, hysterectomy can be very successful in relieving chronic pelvic pain. One study of more than 300 women treated for pelvic pain with hysterectomy found that 74 percent of the women had complete eradication of pain, 21 percent had decreased pain, and only 5 percent had no benefit. Persistent pain after hysterectomy was more likely to occur in women who had nothing identifiably wrong in the pelvic cavity at the time of surgery.

PELVIC INFECTION / PELVIC INFLAMMATORY DISEASE (PID)

Various pathogens (for example, chlamydia and gonorrhea) cause infections. Bacteria in the reproductive organs can cause pelvic infection, and they can enter the reproductive tract either by passing directly through the mucous membranes and surface lining cells of the reproductive tissues in the vagina or by spreading through the blood vessels. Most of the time, pelvic infection is sexually transmitted. However, infection may also occur when there has been pelvic trauma; after pelvic surgery, because the protective mechanisms and integrity of the pelvic organs have been disrupted during surgery; or when an intrauterine device (IUD) has been used for contraception for a long time.

Pelvic inflammatory disease (PID) is an infection in the pelvic area. It can be difficult to diagnose, and other conditions may be misdiagnosed as PID, or vice versa. Abdominal pain can be caused by such other conditions as viral gastroenteritis and appendicitis, for example. A diagnosis of PID is considered if a woman has these symptoms:

- Lower abdominal pain that may vary in severity and location. The pain may be continuous or intermittent, on the right or the left side, bilateral, or in the middle of the abdomen. The pain may radiate to the back or to the legs. Sometimes the pain is not severe and is perceived only as a nagging discomfort.
- Tenderness in the area of the adnexa (ovaries and tubes).
- Tenderness of the cervix when it is moved from side to side at the time of pelvic examination.

Other symptoms and laboratory findings may include

- fever (temperature higher than 101 °F);
- abnormal cervical or vaginal discharge (generally thick, yellowish or green in color);
- elevated white blood cell count; and
- positive cervical culture for *Neisseria gonorrhoeae* (gonorrhea) or *Chlamydia trachomatis* (chlamydia).

The recommended treatment for PID is a broad-spectrum antibiotic. If PID goes untreated, it can cause pelvic adhesions (scarring), blocked fallopian tubes, infertility, and chronic pelvic pain. *Pyosalpinx*, or pus in the tubes, can develop as a result of PID. It is like an abscess and can lead to infertility and chronic pelvic pain. Following absorption of the pus, a tube may remain blocked or retain tubal fluid. This condition, referred to as *hydrosalpinx*, is associated with infertility.

Usually PID is treated very successfully with oral or intravenous antibiotics. If the PID is more severe or resistant, other treatment might include drainage of an abscess within the tube or ovary; surgical removal of infected tissue, such as removal of an infected fallopian tube or ovary; or hysterectomy if the infection cannot be controlled with antibiotics.

With the availability of many effective antibiotics to fight infection, hysterectomy should be used only as a last resort for treating a pelvic infection. Rarely, when a pelvic infection has caused a pelvic abscess that does not respond to intravenous antibiotic therapy, a hysterectomy may be necessary to eliminate the infection. However, it may be possible to treat such an advanced infection by removal of the tubes or the tubes and ovaries, saving the uterus. The uterus may then be able to carry a pregnancy, as described in Chapter 12.

PELVIC CONGESTION SYNDROME (PCS)

This common condition is also referred to as *varicose veins within the pelvis*. It occurs, like varicose veins in the legs, when the valves in the veins don't work properly and blood flows backward. The blood pools, causing the veins to stretch and bulge. Approximately 15 percent of women aged 20 to 50 have PCS. Although it may cause no symptoms, many women with this condition have symptoms such as pain during and after intercourse, pain when standing that often gets worse during the course of a day, abdominal tenderness, backache, painful or otherwise abnormal periods, irritable bladder, and vaginal discharge. Women who have pelvic congestion syndrome are also likely to have varicose veins in their legs.

The syndrome can be diagnosed through ultrasound or laparoscopy, although these tests can miss PCS because the veins decompress when a woman is lying down. A *venography* is a test in which a contrast solution is injected into the veins of the pelvic organs to enhance visualization. Because it can be difficult to diagnose, PCS is often treated incorrectly—as infection, for example.

Hysterectomy is rarely the best treatment for pelvic congestive syndrome. A relatively new procedure, *ovarian vein embolization*, is effective in plugging up the veins through a catheter to block the accumulation of blood (see Chapter 3). Some medications help constrict the veins, or the veins may be tied off surgically. Of course, the symptoms of PCS need to be severe and interfere significantly with a woman's lifestyle to merit hysterectomy.

GYNECOLOGIC CAUSES OF CHRONIC PELVIC PAIN

Endometriosis and adenomyosis are the most commonly diagnosed gynecologic causes of pelvic pain. Endometriosis, found in 30 to 70 percent of women who have chronic pelvic pain, is described in Chapter 4. Adenomyosis is a benign condition that develops most frequently in women over the age of 35. Although in many women it causes no symptoms, it can be painful and even disabling in others. This is one of the conditions for which hysterectomy is sometimes the best and most effective treatment.

Adenomyosis occurs when tissue from the endometrium, the blood-

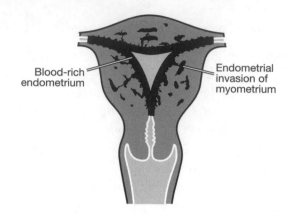

Blood-rich
endometrium

Endometrial
invasion of
myometrium

FIG. 7.1. Adenomyosis. Tissue from the endometrium has extended into the myometrium.

rich inner layer of the uterus, grows into the myometrium, the muscular middle layer of the uterus (fig. 7.1). This tissue, in its new and abnormal location, undergoes typical cyclic growth and bleeding, just as if it were in its normal location within the uterine lining. Swelling and contractions in response to the invading endometrial lining irritate the surrounding muscle tissue. The muscle tissue also grows, and there is a characteristic enlargement of the entire uterus. When a woman with adenomyosis has symptoms, the most common symptom is painful menstrual periods with heavy bleeding.

The cause of adenomyosis is unknown, and it is difficult to determine how common it is because it so often causes no symptoms. Some studies have estimated that 50 percent or more of all women have adenomyosis. It is more likely to occur in a woman who has given birth—80 percent of women with adenomyosis have had children. It also often occurs along with other uterine disorders such as fibroids, endometriosis, and uterine polyps.

Maria was 38, with three children, when she began to experience painful periods (dysmenorrhea). Her heavy menstrual flow dated from shortly after the birth of her last child four years earlier. Her annual pelvic examinations had been normal. Even though an ultrasound examination of the pelvis was negative, because Maria's dysmenorrhea was becoming more severe and lasting longer, her gynecologist recommended a laparoscopy and D&C to seek

an explanation for the pain and heavy bleeding. The only finding was a
slightly enlarged but otherwise normal-appearing uterus. Maria sought a
second opinion from a reproductive endocrinologist, who recommended per-
forming an MRI—which revealed adenomyosis.

Maria had the classic symptoms of adenomyosis: painful and heavy
periods. The dysmenorrhea usually becomes increasingly severe as adenomyosis progresses. Some women with adenomyosis have pain during
intercourse, especially toward the end of the cycle, just before menstruation. If a woman with adenomyosis is examined at this time in her
cycle, her uterus is usually found to be swollen and tender, what gynecologists call a "boggy" uterus.

However, more often women with adenomyosis are symptom-free,
and a pathologist usually makes the diagnosis based on examination of
microscopic sections of a removed uterus. In fact, one of every three hysterectomy specimens is found to contain microscopic evidence of adenomyosis.

If a woman is experiencing pain from adenomyosis, the pain may be
alleviated if she takes oral contraceptives, which prevent ovulation. Anti-
inflammatory medications relieve bleeding and pain by reducing the
production of prostaglandins, chemical substances that are produced in
great quantity by the irritated uterine muscle and may increase pain
by causing uterine contractions. These medications include over-the-
counter (OTC) preparations such as ibuprofen, naproxen sodium, and
many others, as well as prescription drugs. Talk to your gynecologist before using these drugs to treat the symptoms of adenomyosis.

Although symptoms may suggest adenomyosis, to get more information your doctor may want you to have a transvaginal ultrasound examination or magnetic resonance imaging (MRI). The latter distin-
guishes the fine structure of the uterus and is the standard tool for
diagnosing adenomyosis.

When the pain and heavy bleeding of adenomyosis become intolerable and medications fail to relieve these symptoms, we recommend
hysterectomy, which will definitely alleviate these symptoms of adenomyosis. Often the uterus can be removed vaginally. The ovaries
should be conserved whenever possible, especially in young women, because the ovaries are not affected by adenomyosis. When the pain of
adenomyosis is associated with heavy menstrual periods, as frequently

occurs, the endometrial lining should be biopsied before surgery to exclude the possibility of a coexisting malignancy of the endometrium. Women who undergo hysterectomy for adenomyosis can expect to lead lives free of uterine pain following surgery.

PELVIC ADHESIONS

Scarring is often part of the normal healing process; in scarring, fibrous tissue replaces normal tissue. When tissue heals by scarring, adhesions are sometimes formed. Pelvic adhesions are fibrous bands of tissue that connect various organs in the pelvis—large bowel, ovaries, uterus, fallopian tubes, bladder, or peritoneal tissue. The connection may be loose (filmy adhesions), or there may be dense attachments between organs (fig. 7.2).

These attachments can cause pain, especially if they are located in the ovaries or bowel. As the ovaries change shape during the menstrual cycle—for example, as follicles develop and when ovulation occurs— dense scar tissue attaching the ovaries to other organs can place tension on the attached organs or stretch nerve fibers, which can be painful.

Adhesions most often occur as a result of previous surgeries (or as a result of pelvic inflammatory disease or endometriosis). Sometimes inflammation from a pelvic infection or endometriosis causes adhesions to form. Some people have a greater than usual tendency to develop scar tissue when they heal.

The best treatment for pelvic adhesions is to have them removed or cut so that abnormal sites of tension are relaxed. Often adhesions can be treated laparoscopically. Usually a laparoscopic procedure to treat adhesions can be done on an outpatient basis. In many cases, adhesions occur in the first place because of surgery, so we strive to avoid causing more adhesions during further surgery. That's why we recommend laparoscopy to treat adhesions—it is usually less traumatic and causes fewer recurrences than laparotomy, in which the large abdominal incision is more likely to cause trauma to other abdominal tissues. Sometimes, pelvic adhesions are so extensive that it is impossible to identify the borders of the pelvic organs (such as intestinal tract structures or portions of the urinary tract), and the adhesions cannot be cut without causing further damage. When this happens, major surgery to remove

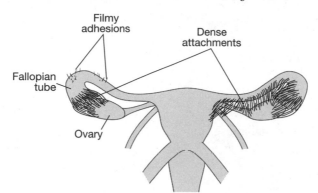

FIG. 7.2. Pelvic adhesions. Adhesions that are loose and filmy are usually less bothersome than dense adhesions, which are more likely to cause pain. Either kind of adhesion may cause infertility.

adhesions may be necessary. A hysterectomy is sometimes the best treatment to relieve the chronic pain associated with adhesions.

Unfortunately, development of pelvic adhesions from the bowel to the peritoneal surface lining the pelvis may result from a hysterectomy. A second surgery, often done by laparoscopy, may be necessary to remove these recurrent pelvic adhesions. The surgical term for removal or cutting of adhesions is lysis of adhesions, or adhesiolysis.

NONGYNECOLOGIC CAUSES OF CHRONIC PELVIC PAIN

Before considering hysterectomy as a treatment for chronic pelvic pain, we evaluate and rule out other possible causes of pelvic pain. Common nongynecologic causes of pelvic pain include

- addiction or substance abuse problem;
- anxiety, especially health-focused anxiety;
- arthritis;
- chronic appendicitis;
- chronic interstitial cystitis (chronic bladder infection);
- depression;
- lumbar disk disease;

- diverticulitis (an intestinal inflammation);
- fibromyalgia;
- functional bowel disease;
- hernia;
- inflammatory bowel disease;
- irritable bowel syndrome;
- physical or sexual abuse; and
- scoliosis (curvature of the spine) and posture-related problems.

MAJOR POINTS

- Pelvic infection can usually be cured with antibiotics. Only rarely is hysterectomy necessary for treatment of PID.
- Adenomyosis is a benign although often painful disorder that involves the growth of endometrial tissue within the uterine muscle. Sometimes hysterectomy is the best treatment for adenomyosis.
- Pelvic adhesions usually can be effectively treated with laparoscopy, but when adhesions are extensive, hysterectomy can be the best solution.
- New adhesions often form following surgery, even after surgery designed to remove adhesions.

CHAPTER 8

Cancer

Agynecologic cancer, particularly uterine cancer, is the most un-
equivocal reason for a woman to have a hysterectomy. But only
about 11 percent of hysterectomies are performed to treat cancer—about 66,000 of the approximately 600,000 hysterectomies done
annually in this country. Fewer than 80,000 cases of gynecologic cancer are diagnosed each year.

There are three major cancers that originate in a woman's reproductive tract: uterine cancer, cervical cancer, and ovarian cancer. Ovarian
cancer does not begin in the uterus, but since its symptoms are subtle
and nonspecific (or not apparent at all), it is often not diagnosed until
late stages, after it has spread to the uterus and beyond. Hysterectomy
is almost always recommended for women with ovarian cancer of any
stage. That is also true for uterine cancer, but women with cervical cancer have a wider range of options.

Cancer consists of more than a hundred different diseases, but there
are many similarities in the way cancers are diagnosed, assessed, and
treated. In this chapter we discuss uterine and cervical cancer and how
and when each of these malignancies can lead to a hysterectomy.

UTERINE CANCER

According to the American Cancer Society, about thirty-six thousand
women develop uterine cancer each year in the United States, making it
the fourth most common cancer in women in this country and the most
common gynecologic malignancy. Thirteen percent of all cancers in
women are uterine cancer.

When we speak of uterine cancer, we are referring to a malignancy that develops in any part of the uterus. Most often it develops in the endometrium; this is also called *endometrial cancer*. Uterine cancer is one of the clearest reasons for a woman to have a hysterectomy.

❦ When Sharon's doctor told her that she'd had an "atypical" finding on her annual Pap test, she felt little concern. With both a mother and a daughter who had had breast cancer, breast cancer was the focus of her cancer fears. Because of her family history, she took tamoxifen, the breast cancer preventive treatment. But endometrial cells had been found in her cervix, and that was abnormal, especially for a postmenopausal woman, as Sharon was.

At her doctor's suggestion, she followed up the Pap test with a colposcopy and endometrial biopsy. She was shocked when the doctor called her and told her she had endometrial cancer—it was not something she had considered. She had none of the risk factors for the disease, except taking tamoxifen. Later her surgeon told her that her cancer had probably started developing before she began taking tamoxifen.

The only treatment option Sharon's doctor suggested was hysterectomy, and it was the only one she wanted to hear. "I wanted to get that whole mess out of there," she remembers. "Just get me home for Christmas," she told her doctor. Diagnosed the first week of December, she had the hysterectomy on the 15th and celebrated the holiday at home with her family. Her abdominal incision was vertical, running from just below her navel to the pubic area, and her uterus, cervix, ovaries, tubes, and some lymph nodes were removed during the operation.

Sharon's recovery was "thankfully uneventful," and she was back at work in a month. Her only problem is that she continues to have symptoms related to hormone deficiency. Because of her risk for breast cancer, she does not wish to take hormone replacement therapy.

Who Develops Uterine Cancer?

Uterine cancer is usually a disease of a woman's later years; approximately 75 percent of all cases are diagnosed in postmenopausal women. The median age for a woman to develop uterine cancer is 61. Most women are very aware of breast cancer, because it gets so much media attention, and cervical cancer, because of Pap testing. But a diagnosis of uterine cancer often comes as a surprise, as it did for Sharon, who was age 50 when she was diagnosed.

The factors that increase a woman's risk for uterine cancer include

- unopposed estrogen use (estrogen replacement therapy, or ERT);
- excess body weight;
- history of endometrial hyperplasia;
- late onset of menopause;
- diabetes;
- hypertension;
- nulliparity (never had children);
- early age at onset of menstruation;
- history of polycystic ovaries; and
- history of breast cancer or ovarian cancer or both.

The first three items on the list are the most potent risk factors, particularly when they occur in combination. Overweight women and those with late onset of menopause should be cautious about using estrogen replacement therapy without the addition of progesterone or a progestin if they haven't had a hysterectomy. The warning, in fact, extends to all women, because the greatest increase in risk with unopposed estrogen therapy applies to women who have no other risk factors for uterine cancer. (Hormone replacement therapy is discussed in Chapter 13.)

A clear relationship exists between atypical endometrial hyperplasia and endometrial cancer. As discussed in Chapter 6, endometrial hyperplasia is related to exposure of the endometrium to prolonged unopposed estrogen—continuous exposure to estrogen, a hormone that causes tissue growth unless its effects are offset to some degree by exposure to progesterone, a hormone that counteracts the growth effects of estrogen on the uterine lining. For a woman with a uterus, taking estrogen alone (for example, as in some regimens of hormone replacement therapy) without combining it with a progesterone-like hormone (progestin) significantly increases the risk of developing endometrial cancer. Because this relationship of "unopposed" estrogen to hyperplasia and endometrial cancer is so well recognized, most regimens of hormone replacement therapy today involve the use of a progesterone-like drug in addition to estrogen.

Unlike menopausal hormone replacement, oral contraceptives have been shown to decrease a woman's risk of developing uterine cancer, probably because they contain the progestin (together with estrogen). Women who have used them for as little as a year have half the risk of developing endometrial cancer as women who have never taken them. This protective effect continues for ten years. Use of oral contraceptives by reproductive-age women is thought to prevent as many as two thousand cases of endometrial cancer each year.

A generation ago, an author writing for the medical journal *Cancer* described a "typical" endometrial cancer patient, listing characteristics that we find still hold true today:

> The typical endometrial cancer patient is an obese, relatively tall postmenopausal woman. She will tend to have a history of short but heavy menstrual periods and some premenstrual breast swelling. Her menopause will have occurred later than in women in the general population. She may have a history of diabetes and hypertension. In one out of three cases she will give a history of spontaneous abortion. In one out of ten instances she will present evidence of goiter or hypothyroidism. If the disease occurs premenopausally, the patient may have a history of irregular menstrual cycles.*

Symptoms

The most common symptom of uterine cancer is abnormal bleeding—a change in your bleeding pattern or bleeding when it ordinarily should not occur. An example of a change in bleeding pattern is prolonged or increased menstrual flow. An example of bleeding when it ordinarily should not occur is between menstrual periods or after menopause. Most postmenopausal bleeding is related to a benign cause. Only one out of five women who experience postmenopausal bleeding has a malignancy of the reproductive tract. However, since three-fourths of all endometrial cancers occur in postmenopausal women, bleeding after menopause requires prompt and thorough attention.

Perimenopause is the one- to two-year interval in a woman's life before her periods cease completely; during this time a woman still has

*E. Wynder, G. Escher, and N. Mantel, "An Epidemiological Investigation of Cancer of the Endometrium." *Cancer* 19 (1966):189.

menstrual periods, but some menopausal symptoms occur, as well. Periods may become less regular and different, often lighter. Because irregularities in menstruation are very common during perimenopause, it is often difficult to determine the significance of bleeding during this transitional interval. A reasonable approach is to accept lighter and less frequent periods as the norm during perimenopause. If bleeding during perimenopause becomes frequent, heavy, or totally irregular, the endometrium should be evaluated by biopsy or dilatation and curettage for the possibility of endometrial cancer or other growths such as fibroids and polyps.

How does your physician decide which procedure to do? The simplest and most direct way to evaluate the endometrium is by endometrial biopsy (see Chapter 2), taking a sample of endometrium for laboratory evaluation. This form of sampling is generally simple, takes little time, and requires no anesthesia. However, there is some dispute about the value of the information it supplies. Although a positive finding indicates a malignancy, a biopsy specimen that shows no evidence of endometrial cancer may not rule out a malignancy because a biopsy samples only a small fragment of tissue, and it may miss the portion of the uterus that contains a malignancy.

We suggest the following guidelines. If your doctor feels that the biopsy specimen has not provided a satisfactory representation of all the tissue that lines the uterine cavity, a dilatation and curettage should be performed (see Chapter 2). If atypical hyperplasia or extensive complex hyperplasia is found on the office biopsy specimen, a D&C also should be done to ensure there are no areas of endometrium that contain cancer cells. If the office biopsy specimen is considered adequate and is interpreted as normal but you continue to experience abnormal bleeding, a D&C should be done as well as a hysteroscopic examination of the cavity of the uterus.

Pelvic ultrasound is another useful diagnostic tool in that it provides specific information about the thickness or regularity of the endometrium. A thickened endometrial stripe (thicker than 5 mm) or an irregular stripe found with ultrasound in a woman who is postmenopausal, especially one who is experiencing bleeding, is an indication for follow-up by hysteroscopy and D&C. (See Chapter 2 for more information on these diagnostic tests.)

Grading and Staging

Uterine cancer is classified in two ways, and these classifications determine treatment possibilities and prognosis. One classification is based on grading the appearance of the cells; the other depends on the degree of extension of the tumor with respect to the uterine muscle. Once endometrial cancer is diagnosed from tissue obtained by a biopsy or D&C, the pathologist assigns a grade from 1 to 3 to the tissue that has been examined. This grade is based on degree of differentiation—the difference between the endometrial cancer cell and normal tissue, and a measure of the maturity and organization of individual cancer cells. Tissue classified as being well differentiated (grade 1) resembles normal endometrium—the closer the resemblance of the cancer cells to the normal endometrium, the better differentiated the cancer. Less differentiated tissue (grades 2 and 3) contains immature endometrial cells, which tend to be arranged in a disorganized manner. A well-differentiated cancer has an excellent prognosis for cure. The less differentiated the tumor, the greater the chance it will have invaded the uterine muscle and spread beyond the uterus itself.

The depth of invasion of the uterine muscle is another important prognostic sign. Cancers that are more superficial and confined to the endometrium have a greater chance for cure. The more deeply a cancer has entered the muscle, the greater the possibility that it has begun to spread farther into or beyond the uterus. The extent of the tumor can be determined only by microscopic examination of the whole uterus, after it has been removed. Poorly differentiated cancers have a higher chance of deep invasion and spread to lymph nodes; cancers that have deeply invaded the wall of the uterus also are more likely to have spread to lymph nodes.

Treatment

Hysterectomy is the mainstay in the treatment of uterine cancer. The need for additional treatment after surgery depends on the findings at the time of the operation—a systematic evaluation called *surgical staging*.

Surgical staging for endometrial cancer is done after a total abdominal hysterectomy along with removal of both tubes and ovaries, as well as an abdominal "wash" to look for cancer cells outside the uterus. After the abdominal incision is made, the abdominal cavity is flushed with a saline solution. This irrigating fluid is then collected in a specimen container and sent to the laboratory to search for abnormal cells under a microscope. The presence of abnormal cells in the fluid of the abdominal cavity indicates that the cancer has spread to the surface of other parts of the abdomen.

At the very beginning of the procedure the surgeon will examine the abdominal organs, including the liver, spleen, and kidneys, and biopsy any suspicious tissue that is found. The surgeon will also remove lymph nodes in the pelvis and surrounding the aorta, the main blood vessel to the heart, and send them to the laboratory for examination.

All removed tissue and fluids are sent to the laboratory, where a pathologist performs a microscopic examination. The pathologist interprets the findings and provides a complete report. This pathological exam is a comprehensive process that makes it possible to classify the extent of the disease and helps to determine whether the surgical procedure was sufficient or if additional treatment is required. The National Cancer Institute and the International Federation of Gynecology and Obstetrics (FIGO) describe the following stages and substages for endometrial cancer:

- STAGE I: The cancer is confined to the corpus, the main body of the uterus. This stage is subdivided into three categories: IA, in which cancer is limited to the endometrium; IB, in which malignant cells are found in the myometrium but in less than half of it; IC, in which cancerous cells have invaded more than half the myometrium.
- STAGE II: The uterine corpus and cervix are involved, but the cancer has not spread beyond the uterus. In Stage IIA, only the glandular cells of the cervix are involved; in IIB, the stromal cells have also been invaded.
- STAGE III: The cancer has spread outside the uterus but is confined to the pelvic area. In Stage IIIA, evidence of cancer is found in the serosa, the outer layer of the uterus, and/or the fallopian tubes and ovaries, and/or the peritoneal wash yields cancer cells. In IIIB, cancer is found in the vagina. In IIIC, cancer is found in lymph nodes, either those in the pelvis or those around the aorta.
- STAGE IV: The cancer has spread beyond the pelvic area. Stage IVA

means the bladder or bowel has been invaded, or both. In Stage IVB, the most serious, the cancer has spread to distant sites in the body, for example, the lungs.

The stage of the cancer largely determines the treatment. Hysterectomy and removal of the tubes and ovaries are usually sufficient treatment for Stage I, when the tumor is limited to the endometrium or penetrates only superficially into the muscle of the uterus. More advanced stages may require postoperative radiation therapy, more extensive surgery, and/or chemotherapy. Women with invasion to the muscle greater than 50 percent usually receive pelvic radiation.

One controversial issue has been whether women who have had endometrial cancer (and hysterectomy) should be given estrogen replacement therapy. Until recently it was thought that estrogen replacement therapy is not a good idea for women who have been treated for endometrial cancer. Several recent clinical studies have determined that estrogen therapy probably poses little risk for women with well-differentiated early stage endometrial cancer. However, these studies are based on small numbers of participants, and the use of estrogen replacement therapy in women who have had endometrial cancer remains controversial. The protective effects of estrogen replacement therapy against osteoporosis in some cases may outweigh the theoretical risk of recurrence of the cancer as a result of hormonal replacement treatment in this specific situation. Osteoporosis is currently being treated with other, nonestrogen drugs such as alendronate and risedronate. Severe menopausal symptoms such as hot flashes and forgetfulness, however, may so significantly interfere with a woman's lifestyle that estrogen treatment may be merited. (See Chapter 13 for a complete discussion of hormone replacement therapy.)

Cervical Cancer

Cancer of the cervix is the second most common cancer among women worldwide (breast cancer is the first). The American Cancer Society estimates that approximately 16,000 new cases of invasive cervical cancer occur each year in the United States, with nearly 5,000 deaths related to this disease. In some countries, the rate of cervical cancer is much higher than in the United States because of less effective screening efforts. The average age of a woman at diagnosis in the United States is 52.2 years.

Cervical cancer is easily detected in its early stages, thanks to the Papanicolaou (Pap) test, a screening test that is usually done when women have gynecologic exams. This test takes a sample—or smear—of cells from a woman's cervix to be examined microscopically. In the decades since the use of Pap smears has become widespread in the United States, the identification of an early stage of cervical cancer and precancerous cervical conditions such as dysplasia has significantly improved, enhancing the curability of cervical cancer and lowering mortality rates from the disease. But not all women get the test regularly, as recommended, and it is not a perfect test. (For a detailed explanation of the Pap test, see Chapter 2 and later in this chapter.)

Who Gets Cervical Cancer?

Cervical cancer is twice as common among African American and Hispanic American women compared with white women, and the incidence is even higher for Native Americans. One group with a less than average risk is Jewish women, as demonstrated by population studies in Israel and the United States. Possible explanations for this are periods of sexual abstinence among Orthodox Jews during and after menstruation, male circumcision, and possible undetermined genetic factors. There is also a lower incidence of cervical cancer among Muslim and Amish women.

In addition to ethnicity, sexual history is a factor related to a woman's chances of developing cervical cancer. A woman who first has intercourse before she is 16 years old is twice as likely to develop cervical cancer as a woman who had her first intercourse after the age of 20. Having multiple sexual partners throughout a woman's lifetime also increases the risk of developing cervical cancer. As far back as the mid-nineteenth century, it was observed that cervical cancer was rarely seen among nuns, although other cancers of the reproductive tract (for example, endometrial cancer) were. This observation has been borne out by a number of studies of nuns in various religious communities throughout the world.

The incidence, prevalence, and mortality of cervical cancer have also been correlated with socioeconomic level.

Cervical cancer is also associated with cigarette smoking. Smokers have twice the risk of developing the disease as nonsmokers. The longer a woman smokes and the more heavily she smokes, the greater her risk of cervical cancer.

Women whose immune systems are suppressed (for example, women who have had kidney or other organ transplants and are on immune-system-suppressing drugs, or women infected with human immuno-deficiency virus [HIV]) are at increased risk for cervical cancer. These women also tend to have more rapidly progressing tumors.

All these observations notwithstanding, the single most important factor in the development of cervical cancer is a virus called *human papilloma virus* (HPV). In a woman with cervical cancer, HPV can be found in the cervical epithelial tissue, the thin surface layer that in the cervix is also known as squamous cells. HPV—actually a group of more than eighty types of viruses—is sexually transmitted. Some types of HPVs have been found to cause genital warts, but less than half of the HPV types infect the genital tract. The specific types most often associated with cervical cancer are HPV-16, HPV-18, HPV-31, and HPV-45. DNA of the first three types has been found in more than 80 percent of cervical cancers.

Cancer is not usually thought of as a sexually transmitted disease, but cervical cancer can be classified as one because of the role of HPV. We have seen that women with multiple sexual partners are at increased risk of developing cervical cancer. Some studies have also found that husbands of women with cervical cancer have had more sexual partners than those whose wives do not have cervical cancer. Women who have had other sexually transmitted diseases, including syphilis and gonorrhea, often also have HPV.

Results of the Pap Smear

About fifty million Pap tests are performed each year in the United States. With a laboratory screening test as effective and inexpensive as the Pap smear, it is hard to understand why not all women have Pap smears at regular intervals from one to three years. One of the most important aspects of the Pap test is that it detects not only cancer but also precancerous conditions. Thus, by alerting a woman and her physician to the need to continue close surveillance and to initiate appropriate treatment, this test can prevent cancer. It is one of the most successful screening devices in medical history. Unfortunately, it is not foolproof, and sometimes a Pap smear misses detecting a cervical cancer. The procedure for performing a Pap test is described in Chapter 2.

Originally Pap smears were graded according to five classes designated by Roman numerals. Classes I and II meant benign cells, Class III indicated moderate or severe dysplasia, Class IV suggested carcinoma in situ (see below), and Class V indicated invasive cervical cancer. Since the original work of Papanicolaou and his colleagues, the procedure has been refined, and new classification systems for interpreting the smears are now in place. The modern classification system, known as the Bethesda system, divides abnormal cervical cells into three main categories:

- *ASCUS,* which is an acronym for *atypical squamous cells of undetermined significance.* ASCUS is the most common abnormality, found in from 2 to 11 percent of all Pap smears reported in this country. How it is treated depends on other factors, but follow-up is important for anyone who is diagnosed with ASCUS. The latest classification, the Bethesda System 2001, subdivided ASCUS into two categories: ASC-US (atypical squamous cells—undetermined significance) and ASC-H (cannot exclude HSIL, explained below). Atypical glandular cells (AGC) may also be identified.
- *LSIL,* or *low-grade squamous intraepithelial lesion.* The word *lesion* refers to an area of abnormal tissue, and *intraepithelial* means that the abnormal cells are present only in the surface layer of cells. *Low-grade* indicates early changes in the size and shape of cells.
- *HSIL,* or *high-grade squamous intraepithelial lesion. High-grade* means that there are more marked changes in the size and shape of the abnormal (precancerous) cells and they look very different from normal cells.

ASCUS and LSIL are considered relatively mild abnormalities, but HSIL is more serious with a greater likelihood of progressing to invasive cancer. LSIL would most likely correspond to Class II and HSIL to Classes III and IV in the earlier classification system.

Dysplasia and *cervical intraepithelial neoplasia* (CIN) are other terms that describe abnormal cells that yield a positive Pap result. Dysplastic cells look abnormal under the microscope, but they do not invade nearby healthy tissue. Dysplasia is classified as mild, moderate, or severe, depending on the degree of abnormality and the proportion of the tissue occupied by the abnormal cells.

Cervical intraepithelial neoplasia is the proliferation of immature cervical squamous cells on the surface tissue without penetration into or through the underlying membrane. *Neoplasia* means an abnormal new growth of cells, and *intraepithelial* refers to the surface layers. CIN is divided into three subclasses, numbered 1 to 3, to describe how much of the thickness of the lining of the cervix contains abnormal cells. The risk of progression of CIN to invasive cervical cancer is directly related to the grade of the lesion, the degree of malignant features in the tissue. A high-grade lesion is more serious than a low-grade lesion.

The classification of a Pap smear is very important in determining what additional tests are necessary for a definitive diagnosis. The Pap smear is a screening test that samples superficial cells, and as such it can miss markedly abnormal cells if the mouth of the cervix (ectocervix) and cervical canal (endocervix) are not sampled in their entirety or if there is a lesion that fails to shed abnormal cells from its surface. Sampling errors are reduced when the physician uses a cytobrush instead of a swab to obtain the sample and when liquid-based Pap smear methods are used.

It is difficult for a patient to evaluate the quality of a cytology laboratory that reviews Pap smears. Some insurance companies require Pap smears to be sent to a lab with which they have a contract. The contract may go to a lab with the best price and not the best quality of interpretation. It is in your best interest to ask your gynecologist about the quality of the lab.

What If It Is Cancer?

When cancer cells are clearly identified in a Pap smear, the Bethesda Classification System reports them as cancer. Cancer of the cervix usually originates from the squamous cells of the cervix growing from the area of the cervix where the ectocervical tissue (outer tissue covered by squamous mucosa) meets the cervical canal (inner tissue lined by glandular cells). This area is known as the *transformation zone*. The name is accurate—the tissue at this site, the squamous cellular lining, is constantly undergoing changes in form and structure, a phenomenon known as *squamous metaplasia* (fig. 8.1).

Most cancers of the cervix begin as *preinvasive cancer*, or *intraep-*

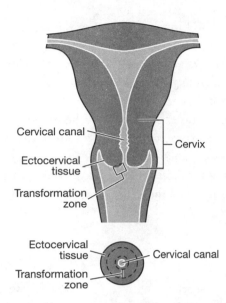

FIG. 8.1. The parts of the cervix, including the transformation zone, where cervical cancer originates. The transformation zone is the area where the outer cervical tissue (ectocervix) and tissue lining the cervical canal (endocervical tissue) meet.

ithelial neoplasia, which does not penetrate the membrane beneath it. This is also called *carcinoma in situ.* The earliest evidence of spread of the cancer, or invasion, is referred to as *microinvasion.* At this stage, the lesion invades the underlying tissue to a small depth (3 mm or less) below the base of the epithelial cells. With deeper invasion, the tumor may involve blood vessels and lymphatic tissue.

When cervical cancer spreads, it does so by extending directly through the underlying membrane. It progressively reaches adjacent organs such as the bladder and rectum or enters lymph channels, through which it spreads to the lymph nodes, which drain the nearby organs. Cervical cancer also extends upward and downward to areas adjacent to the cervix—upward to the endometrium or downward to the upper portion of the vagina. It can also grow laterally through the cervix to the side walls of the pelvis, forward to the base of the bladder, or backward to the rectum. Invasion into blood vessels leads to distant spread (metastases), and spread into lymphatic channels leads to metastases in the pelvic lymph nodes.

Progression of CIN to invasive cancer takes several years, and some early lesions may never progress—they sometimes even disappear without treatment. Women with impaired immunity (for example, from HIV infection or renal transplant) are at greatest risk for progression. Estimates show that in women with CIN, 60 percent of the time the lesion will get better on its own; 10 percent of the time it will progress to CIN II; and 1 percent of women with CIN will progress to invasive cancer. The remainder stay stable, with neither regression nor progression.

Although cervical cancer is often discovered with a Pap smear before there are any symptoms, the disease can cause symptoms, particularly if it has begun to spread.

Symptoms

The symptoms associated with cervical cancer include abnormal vaginal bleeding or vaginal discharge. Abnormal bleeding can occur in several ways: as spotting or bleeding between periods, spotting after intercourse, or prolonged and/or heavy menstrual flow. Discharge may be bloody, yellow or brown in color, and may be associated with an unpleasant odor, which usually reflects degeneration of malignant tissue.

Pain only occurs when cervical cancer has spread to other parts of the body or if the tumor has undergone *necrosis* (breakdown). If the cancer has spread to the bladder or rectum, it also can cause symptoms related to these organs such as blood in the urine or rectal bleeding.

Diagnosis and Treatment

You should be certain that you receive notification about the report on your Pap smear. If you receive a report of an abnormal finding on a Pap smear, or if your doctor observes anything abnormal in the internal examination, it means you need a biopsy to obtain further information. If you are diagnosed with ASCUS, we recommend having the Pap smear repeated. If there is any indication of inflammation, it's a good idea to treat the cervical or vaginal infection before the smear is repeated. In women who are menopausal and are not receiving hormone replacement therapy, before repeating the Pap smear we recommend treatment for several weeks with estrogen, using a vaginal insert or cream or systemic pill or patch. The estrogen supports the growth of normal tissue; lack of estrogen may have led to cellular changes that caused the ASCUS finding.

If two or more Pap smears identify ASCUS, or if a woman with ASCUS has other risk factors for cervical cancer (for example, HIV, HPV, multiple sexual partners), we recommend colposcopy. Colposcopy is also recommended for women with ASCUS who have any other laboratory or clinical findings that suggest the possibility of a serious cervical lesion.

Colposcopy (described in detail in Chapter 2) allows examination of the cervix through a stereoscopic binocular microscope. The magnification provided by this treatment allows the examiner to observe characteristics of the tissue that may be responsible for the abnormal Pap smear. This tissue may be biopsied during the procedure, and cells are also collected from the central internal canal of the cervix (endocervical canal) using a curette. All the sampled material is sent to a pathology laboratory for evaluation.

Two further diagnostic procedures can also serve as treatment—LEEP and cervical conization. *Loop electrosurgical excision* of the cervix (LEEP) is a more extensive biopsy, used when the colposcopy does not explain the abnormal cells found on the Pap smear or when endocervical curettings reveal intraepithelial cancer. LEEP is performed when there is Pap smear or colposcopic evidence of a high-grade squamous lesion (HSIL) or a persistent diagnosis of a low-grade squamous lesion (LSIL), especially in a woman at high risk for cervical cancer. It is usually done in the doctor's office, under local anesthesia. It removes the transformation zone of the cervix (the area of the cervix where cancer is most likely to develop) and any malignancy that may be there (fig. 8.2).

Cervical conization is a more extensive form of cervical biopsy than LEEP. It is done in an operating room under anesthesia. In this procedure the doctor removes the transformation zone of the cervix in the shape of a cone. The widest portion of the cone is around the ectocervix, where the cervix meets the vagina. The cone shape tapers as it begins to go up the cervical canal. It has the advantage (unlike LEEP) of not electrocauterizing residual tissue, which could interfere with interpretation of future Pap smears (fig. 8.3).

We recommend that cervical conization or LEEP be used under any of the following circumstances:

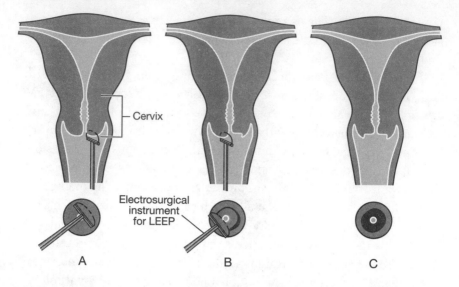

Cervix

Electrosurgical
instrument
for LEEP

A   B   C

FIG. 8.2. LEEP procedure, in which tissue in the transformation zone of the cervix is removed using an electrosurgical loop. *A*. The loop is applied to the transformation zone. *B*. The loop removes the entire transformation zone in a circular fashion. *C*. Appearance of the cervix (now lacking the transformation zone) after the LEEP procedure. The top views show the entire uterus and the bottom views show the cervix in a direct view.

- If colposcopy does not identify the area that is causing the abnormal Pap smear
- If colposcopic biopsy results do not adequately explain the reason for abnormal cells found on the Pap smear, indicating that they may be coming from a lesion higher up in the canal than can be visually identified
- If there is extension of atypical tissue into the cervical canal
- If areas of microscopic invasion (microinvasive cancer) are found on the cervical biopsy
- If tissue obtained by endocervical curettage reveals cervical intraepithelial neoplasia

Treatment of cervical intraepithelial neoplasia using loop electrosurgical excision of the cervix or conization is more common today than it was in years past, and it is used especially in women who wish to pre-

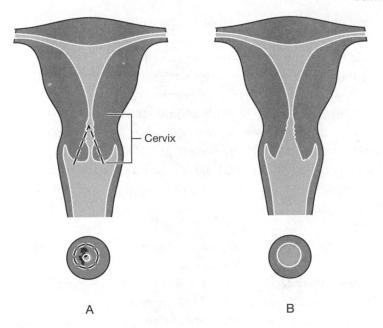

FIG. 8.3. Cervical conization, in which a knife is used to remove the trans-formation zone of the cervix and underlying tissue in the shape of a cone. *A.* Indicates the cone of tissue that will be removed from the cervix. *B.* The appearance of the cervix after removal of tissue in a cervical conization.

serve their uterus and avoid hysterectomy. Pregnancy and childbear-ing are definitely possible following conservative treatment of intra-epithelial cervical cancer. When the cervical lesion is at the dysplasia stage, it can be cut out along with a sizable amount of tissue; this is con-sidered state-of-the-art management when a woman wishes to retain her uterus. However, if there is any evidence that the cervical cancer has become invasive—that is, spread beyond its original site—hysterectomy is usually the best treatment.

Hysterectomy and Other Treatment Options

Although hysterectomy is the usual treatment for cervical cancer, there are other treatment options for both early and late stages of this disease.

The carbon dioxide laser is one way of vaporizing tissue. It should be used only for treatment of early stage disease because no tissue remains for pathologic examination with this procedure. With the carbon dioxide laser, after biopsies are taken, the laser beam is used to destroy small abnormal areas of the cervix without destroying normal tissue.

Cryosurgery may also be used for the treatment of cervical dysplasia and carcinoma in situ. In this procedure liquid nitrogen is used to create a cold surface on an instrument that is applied directly to the cervix and causes destruction by freezing of the abnormal cervical areas. The main disadvantage of this method is that no cervical tissue is available for pathologic evaluation to determine whether the entire area of abnormality has been destroyed by freezing. Thus, follow-up with repeat Pap smears is critical.

Besides LEEP and cervical conization, cervical intraepithelial neoplasia can be treated with carbon dioxide laser or cryosurgery, once it has been definitively shown that there is no invasive cancer. These methods either remove or destroy the transformation zone, the portion of the cervix where cancer grows. We emphasize, however, that LEEP, carbon dioxide laser, and cryosurgery should be used to treat CIN *only* when the lesion is completely visualized by colposcopic examination; if not, conization of the cervix should be done. The main advantage of the other forms of therapy is that they can be done without general anesthesia, on an outpatient basis.

After treatment of CIN, we recommend Pap smears at three-month intervals. After one year, if all Pap smears are negative, an annual Pap smear is sufficient for continued monitoring.

When the cancer is invasive, treatment choices depend on the extent and location of the spread of the malignancy. The International Federation of Gynecology and Obstetrics recognizes a staging system for cervical cancer similar to the one we described for endometrial cancer.

Staging is a very important concept in understanding the treatment of cervical cancer. The staging system is based on what your doctor finds in the clinical exam, X-ray studies, tissue sampling, proctoscopy, and cystoscopy. During the clinical exam, the areas around the involved cervix are viewed and examined manually for evidence of extension beyond the cervix. Proctoscopy (viewing the rectal tissue through an endoscope inserted in the rectum) and cystoscopy (viewing the bladder lining through a scope inserted through the urethra) allow detection of advancement of the cancer into the rectum or bladder, respectively.

The International Federation of Gynecology and Obstetrics (FIGO) staging system for cervical cancer is as follows:

- Stage 0 is noninvasive. Dysplasia and CIN are classified as Stage 0.
- Stage I means the cancer is confined to the cervix. Stage IA can only be seen microscopically; if malignant areas are visible upon visual exam, it is stage IB. Further subclassifications into IA1, IA2, IB1, and IB2 refer to the size of the lesion, ranging from 5 mm deep by 7 mm wide (IA1) to larger than 4 cm (IB2).
- Stage II means the cancer has spread beyond the cervix to the vagina, but not to the pelvic wall. IIA indicates that there is no involvement of the parametrium, the connective tissues of the pelvic floor that surround and are adjacent to the uterus; IIB means there is parametrial involvement.
- In Stage III, the tumor has spread to the pelvic wall or to the lower third of the vagina. IIIA means it is confined to the vagina; IIIB means it has extended to the pelvic wall.
- In Stage IV, the cancer has spread beyond the pelvis. IVA refers to spread to adjacent organs such as the bladder or rectum; IVB to more distant spread.

Surgery and radiation are the two approaches most often used to treat invasive cervical cancer. Surgical treatment for Stage IA, early invasive cancer, is usually a simple or modified radical hysterectomy. For women with Stage IA2, we also take a sampling of the pelvic lymph nodes, so that the nodes can be microscopically examined for any trace of cancer. Younger women with Stage IA may wish to maintain their fertility; if so, they are sometimes given the option of a cervical conization, although this procedure does carry a slight risk of incomplete treatment if the cancer has spread to lymph nodes.

Women with Stages IB1, IB2, and IIA are usually given the option of surgery or radiation. The surgical procedure recommended for these lesions is radical hysterectomy with removal of pelvic lymph nodes. (The radical hysterectomy is described in Chapter 11.) Survival rates for women with these early stages of cervical cancer are comparable after surgery or radiation. For women with an ovarian tumor or a history of inflammatory bowel disease or pelvic inflammatory disease, surgery is usually the preferred treatment, rather than radiation.

Both surgery and radiation have a number of advantages and disadvantages, and you will want to review these carefully with your doctor and your family before making treatment decisions. Even with the same stage of disease, surgery might be right for one woman, radiation for another. It is a very personal decision. To guide you in making your decision, we list the following advantages and disadvantages. Keep in mind that this book is a guide to hysterectomy and not a comprehensive discussion of cervical cancer, and we present here only a brief overview of these issues.

Advantages of surgery:

- Preservation of ovaries and ovarian function
- Maintenance of the quality of vaginal tissues
- Reduced incidence of long-term side effects
- Opportunities for a complete evaluation of pelvic and abdominal structures by direct observation at the time of surgery

Possible complications of surgery:

- Shortening of the vagina
- Formation of a fistula (a passageway) between the vagina and the urinary tract or bowel shortly after surgery
- Infection, wound breakdown, reaction to anesthesia, or injury to the bladder, bowel, or major blood vessels

Fistulous connections with the vagina can usually be repaired surgically. Vaginal shortening is reversible and will occur to some extent after resumption of intercourse.

Advantages of radiation therapy:

- Reduced hospitalization (depending on what type of radiation therapy is used)
- No need for general anesthesia or surgical procedures

Possible complications of radiation therapy:

- Loss of ovarian function (because radiation affects the ovaries)
- Atrophic changes and fibrosis (thickening with scar tissue and less pliable vaginal tissues), with impairment or loss of sexual function

- Formation of a fistula between the vagina and the urinary tract or bowel several years after surgery because of blood vessel changes and fibrosis

For more advanced stages of invasive cervical cancer (Stages IIB, III, IV), radiation therapy is usually preferred. Once the cancer has spread beyond the cervix, there is no survival benefit to removing the cervix and uterus, and their removal would subject a woman to unnecessary surgery. Radiation can be administered both externally and through the vagina.

Major Points

- Cancer is the most compelling reason for a woman to have a hysterectomy. The three major gynecologic cancers for which hysterectomy is used are uterine, cervical, and ovarian.
- Atypical endometrial hyperplasia precedes and is associated with development of endometrial cancer if left untreated. Abnormal uterine bleeding and postmenopausal bleeding are the most common symptoms of uterine cancer, and they should be evaluated promptly.
- HPV infection of the cervix is a sexually transmitted disease that may cause cervical cancer.
- The Pap test detects precancerous cervical abnormalities and cervical cancer. Dysplasia and noninvasive cancer can be treated with various methods, but hysterectomy or radiation is recommended for any invasive cervical cancer that has not spread beyond the cervix.

Part III

SURGERY

Once you have made the decision to have a hysterectomy, you can focus on the specific preparations necessary for surgery and then on the surgery itself. Again, we emphasize the importance of finding out everything you want to know about the procedure. Having this information will ease your personal concerns, help you to make the best preparations possible, and allow you to be a partner with your doctor in any decisions that need to be made.

In this section, we tell you how to prepare for a hysterectomy, we provide an overview of the surgery, and then we explain in detail each of the different surgical approaches to hysterectomy.

CHAPTER 9

What You Need to Know to Prepare for a Hysterectomy

Many of our patients tell us they feel great relief when they make the decision to have a hysterectomy. Many have suffered years of pain and discomfort and have tried a succession of other treatment options, with varying degrees of success and failure. Finally, they can look forward to moving on from that. Once the decision about hysterectomy is made, of course, other issues have to be faced and other decisions made.

Hysterectomy is almost always an elective procedure—one that a woman chooses to undergo and that can, to a certain extent, be scheduled at her convenience. Some medical conditions must be treated more urgently than others, but usually there is time for a woman to reflect and to gather as much information as she needs about what she is going to experience.

℃ *The days are gone when you could go to your doctor and say, "This hurts. Fix me," Beverly mused after her hysterectomy. "You have to take responsibility for your own treatment. That's one thing I learned from my hysterectomy."*

Keep in mind that nearly everyone feels somewhat anxious as he or she prepares for major surgery, but don't talk yourself into ignoring any questions you have. All your questions are important and need to be answered. Getting good answers to your concerns will generally help ease your anxieties.

FINDING THE RIGHT DOCTOR

One way to decrease the stress of major surgery is to make sure you get the best medical care you can find. We know it can be difficult to assess the quality of medical and surgical care, and it also can be uncomfortable to ask your doctor specific questions about how much experience and training he has. But gynecology is one of the few medical fields in which the person who provides your routine care is usually the person who will do your surgery. So if you have an ongoing and trusting relationship with your gynecologist, you may already be satisfied that your doctor is not only well trained and technically proficient but also able to anticipate and answer your questions.

❦ "I don't know why I trusted my doctor, but I did," said Julie, who had been to a number of doctors whom she didn't trust in her years of dealing with pelvic pain and abnormal bleeding. "With this doctor, there was something about her—her demeanor, her confidence, her patience with my husband. It all came together."

If you haven't known your gynecologist for long, you can make judgments based on the doctor's willingness to listen and her ability to answer your questions in an understandable way. You can get information about your physician's training from the American Board of Medical Specialties or through your county medical society. Most states have listings of lawsuits that have been filed against physicians, and that information might be of interest. If you are looking for a physician to do your surgery and don't know where to turn, you might start at the gynecology department of a large academic medical center—every state has at least one. And one of the most time-honored ways of finding a physician is also one of the best—ask your relatives, friends, or co-workers if they know a doctor they would recommend.

Hysterectomy has psychological as well as physical consequences, so you should also feel comfortable that your doctor is sensitive and experienced in dealing with the psychological consequences of treating gynecologic disorders. We try to address the concerns of the women we treat by listening to them, caring about them, and treating them with respect. As part of that respect, we endorse a policy for gynecologists first to talk with a woman while she is clothed rather than after she has already donned a gown. We make ourselves accessible, providing phone numbers where we can be reached and telling our patients not to hesitate to call. We always ask them whether they have questions for us. We try to be sensitive to the tone of a woman's voice as an indication of her underlying fears and concerns. In order to have a context for the medical care we provide, we take an interest in aspects of the lives of the women we treat beyond the strictly medical.

One question that many women will have, particularly in a teaching hospital, is who will actually do the surgery. Every woman has the right to expect that her doctor will be in the operating room, organizing the surgical team, supervising the procedure, and making necessary decisions —even if a resident makes incisions or puts in the sutures.

IMPACT OF HYSTERECTOMY

To give you an idea of how different operations rank in seriousness, we will describe a hospital's surgical classification system, which divides surgical procedures into five categories. Category 1 refers to the least invasive types of surgery, such as a D&C; category 5, which includes open-heart surgery and liver transplantation, contains the most complex types of surgical procedures. Hysterectomy falls right in the middle, in category 3.

The impact of a surgery, however, may go beyond its classification. Removal of a uterus has far greater emotional significance on the patient than removal of an appendix or gallbladder or a joint replacement. Any surgical procedure on the female reproductive tract can have far-reaching implications that transcend a successful outcome. This is especially true of hysterectomy. The prospects of this surgery threaten your control over your own body and may affect your sexuality. Many women speak of the fear of feeling "less like a woman" after hysterectomy. It is important to be emotionally as well as physically ready for the surgery. It's not always easy.

After years of suffering severe and painful symptoms from fibroids, Stephanie made the decision to have a hysterectomy. Even though she felt certain this was the best course to take, she was frightened and nervous. She spent the night before the surgery at a hotel across the street from the hospital and couldn't stop thinking about all the risks associated with anesthesia and what could go wrong after surgery.

Rebecca also had fibroids and had tried for years to become pregnant but never conceived. Emotionally, she found the hysterectomy decision to be "gut-wrenching." Once her surgery was scheduled, she couldn't bear to see a woman with a baby. The finality of what she was going to do was nearly overwhelming.

When her doctor told her he thought she should have a hysterectomy, Leslie read every book she could find on the subject and was alarmed by what she read. She was terrified of the surgery—afraid of being cut, afraid of anesthesia, afraid of not being in control. But she trusted her doctor, and when he recommended hysterectomy, she knew she should put it off no longer.

Here are some of the important questions a woman must address with her doctor as the decision is made to have a hysterectomy:

- Is my general health good enough for me to undergo surgery?
- Will the surgical procedure impair my future health in any way?
- What approach will be taken—vaginal, abdominal, or laparoscopic?
- Will it be necessary for my ovaries to be removed?
- Will it be necessary for my cervix to be removed?

Information to help you explore these questions is provided in this part of our book.

Getting Down to Specifics

Once you are satisfied that hysterectomy is the best answer to your medical problem and you have a general idea about the type of procedure that will work best for you and the extent of surgery you will need, you will probably have more questions about details of the surgery and what it will mean for your life:

- Where will the incision be located and what will the scar look like?
- How long will the surgery take?

- What type of anesthesia will be used and how will I react to it?
- What are the possible risks and complications of the surgery and the anesthesia?
- Who will be my anesthesiologist? Will we meet and talk before my surgery?
- How will I feel immediately after surgery?
- What activities can I do after surgery?
- How long will I remain in the hospital?
- When can I resume all my usual activities? Will I be able to resume my normal lifestyle?
- When can I resume sexual activity? Will I notice any difference in sexual function?
- Will my hormone balance change after surgery?
- What will my doctor do if she finds something unexpected?
- What is the chance that I will need further surgery?

For your own well-being, it is important to have a complete discussion of details such as these with your doctor, so he or she understands your concerns and you understand what is going to occur during and after surgery. The answers your doctor provides will almost certainly give you a more positive attitude about surgery. We find that the women who do best physically and psychologically are those who are well informed about what to expect and have a positive attitude about the operation. In fact, there is every reason to be positive—from the surgeon's point of view, the hysterectomy procedure is a relatively simple one, and contemporary medical and surgical techniques virtually assure a successful outcome. (Some of the questions listed above are addressed directly in Chapter 10.)

THE PREOPERATIVE EVALUATION

Different medical centers have different specific recommendations or requirements for preoperative laboratory screening, especially for healthy women, but every woman must have a complete physical assessment within a month before surgery. This assessment includes a general physical examination by your gynecologist or primary care physician. The examination should be a full physical: blood pressure, weight, pulse rate, respiration rate, listening to your lungs and heart, examining your breasts, checking your abdomen for any enlargements of the internal abdominal organs or pelvic organs. If you haven't had a mammogram and Pap smear in the past year, you may need to get these done, and your doctor may also request blood counts and blood chemistries as well as an electrocardiogram.

Your gynecologist will perform a complete pelvic examination, including a rectal examination, to assess the size and location of the uterus and other organs in the pelvis. This exam will help your gynecologist choose the best procedure to treat your problem. If an abdominal incision is going to be used, the pelvic examination also helps the gynecologist choose the type of incision—midline (vertical) or transverse (horizontal)—that is best for your surgery. If your gynecologist is not going to perform the surgery, then the surgeon who will perform the surgery will examine you to obtain information to help make these decisions.

The physical examination and laboratory tests are also necessary to rule out any underlying medical problems that could complicate surgery, to determine that your general physical condition is healthy enough for you to undergo the operation, and to identify any specific risks from anesthesia and surgery. If a disorder is found, it needs to be treated appropriately or, if treatment isn't necessary, at least the surgeon and anesthesiologist should be alerted to potential medical problems that could arise during surgery or while you are recuperating.

Potential complicating conditions include hypertension (high blood pressure), heart disease, epilepsy, diabetes, and asthma. If you have valvular heart disease (for example, a significant heart murmur or mitral valve prolapse), you should be treated with an antibiotic at the time of surgery to reduce risk of infection to your heart valve. Diabetes should be treated or, if very mild, at least noted so that diet and intravenous fluids during the hospitalization can be adjusted to meet your dietary needs. If you have epilepsy, you should take antiseizure medications. Women with asthma require specialized anesthetic approaches.

At times, the disorder to be considered preoperatively will be the same disorder that is making surgery necessary in the first place. For example, a woman who is having a hysterectomy to treat uterine fibroids that cause heavy menstrual or irregular uterine bleeding may be anemic (low hematocrit and red blood cell count). If you have severe anemia, it is important that it be treated prior to surgery because the surgery can cause additional blood loss. Starting out with normal hemoglobin (red blood cell level) provides an important margin of safety and lessens the chance of needing a blood transfusion during surgery. Sometimes it is impossible to correct an anemia medically before surgery because the bleeding is life-threatening. In that case, a blood transfusion is usually given prior to surgery to bring the blood count up to acceptable levels to reduce surgical risk. (For more information about blood transfusions, see below.)

Sometimes the preoperative evaluation will identify a condition that may take precedence in treatment before the hysterectomy. An example is a suspicious breast lump. Any finding like this needs thorough evaluation because treatment of a malignancy of another organ almost certainly will take priority over an elective hysterectomy. Likewise, if there is an abnormal Pap smear, follow-up studies should be done before surgery, unless the reason for the hysterectomy is cervical cancer.

The Pap smear helps determine if there is a cervical abnormality, which might change the surgical approach or procedure. On rare occasions, even with adequate screening, cervical cancer remains undiagnosed and is found only when the pathologist looks at the tissue that was removed during surgery. If cervical cancer has gone undiagnosed until after surgery, it is possible that the type of hysterectomy that was performed was not extensive enough to treat the cervical cancer adequately. It is much better to know about this problem in advance so that the most effective type of procedure can be performed. Having a normal Pap smear close to the time of the hysterectomy is not a guarantee, but it reduces the chance of undergoing a hysterectomy and learning after the surgery that cervical cancer was found and further gynecologic treatment is necessary. If you have irregular vaginal bleeding that has not been evaluated, you should tell your doctor about it so that appropriate tests can be done. Sometimes abnormal bleeding is the only sign of abnormal cervical or endometrial cells (see Chapters 6 and 8).

Part of preparing for surgery is telling your doctor about all the medications you are taking. Provide a comprehensive list of prescription *and* nonprescription drugs. Tell your doctor about diuretics, blood pressure medications, sedatives, steroids, antidepressants, antiarthritis drugs, and anything else you take. Some over-the-counter drugs such as St. John's wort may interact with anesthetic medication or may interfere with your body's metabolism of anesthetics, and this situation must be taken into account. Also make sure that the doctor knows of any allergy or hypersensitivity you have to specific medications.

Usually you will continue your medications, but there are some exceptions. Aspirin is an example of a widely used medication that should be stopped ten days to two weeks before surgery, unless it is being given to prevent formation of blood clots (for example, in a woman with carotid artery disease). Aspirin acts on the blood platelets to prevent the body's normal clotting mechanisms, and its continued use up to the time of surgery could lead to excessive bleeding during the operation.

Urinary Studies

If you have urinary symptoms, your doctor may order a urinalysis or a urine culture (or both) to check for a urinary tract infection. If you have noticed involuntary leakage of urine (urinary incontinence), you should alert your doctor to this symptom. Involuntary loss of urine is sometimes related to anatomic changes at the bladder neck. Urinary stress incontinence is the most common type of urinary incontinence, occurring in up to 20 percent of women. Stress incontinence is the inadvertent loss of urine that occurs when there is an increase in intra-abdominal pressure, such as when you sneeze, cough, laugh, or exercise. It is more likely to happen when the bladder is full and happens more frequently and inconveniently when the normal mechanism of the bladder and urethra is impaired. Often stress incontinence is also associated with genitourinary prolapse, a relaxation and "dropping" of the pelvic or urinary organs (or both).

A cystometrogram is a study to evaluate urinary incontinence. During this test the pressure and volume relationships of the bladder are measured as the bladder is filled with fluid (generally sterile water) or gas (usually carbon dioxide). This test helps determine the cause of the urinary incontinence and indicates whether surgical correction could treat the problem. Surgical correction of urinary incontinence can often be done at the same time as the hysterectomy, simultaneously correcting the urinary stress incontinence and treating the problem for which the hysterectomy is being done.

Endometrial Biopsy

An endometrial biopsy should be done prior to hysterectomy if you have had any abnormal uterine bleeding, especially if you are near menopause or beyond (see Chapter 2). Identifying an endometrial abnormality prior to surgery might affect the choice of surgical approach or type of procedure to be done.

Other Recommended Laboratory Tests

For women with certain medical conditions, specific laboratory tests are recommended before anesthesia and surgery.

- Electrocardiogram—for women over 50, with hypertension, current or past heart disease, peripheral vascular disease, diabetes, or renal, thyroid, or other metabolic disease.
- Chest X-ray—for women with lung disease; for women with chronic lung disease, an X-ray is recommended if there has been a change of symptoms or an acute episode in the previous six months.
- Electrolytes, blood urea nitrogen (BUN), creatinine—for women with kidney disease or adrenal or thyroid disorders or for women who have had diuretic therapy or chemotherapy within the previous six months.
- Micro-urinalysis—for women with diabetes, kidney disease, genital or urinary infection within the previous three months or any metabolic disorder involving permanent kidney dysfunction.
- Complete blood count—for women with blood-related disorders, cancer, kidney failure, history of any recent (within one month) infection; or for women who have had chemotherapy within the previous six months. This test evaluates several components of blood including white blood cell count and platelet count in addition to the hemoglobin level.
- Coagulation studies—for women with a history of excessive bleeding or anticoagulation therapy.

PREPARING FOR A BLOOD TRANSFUSION

Sometimes during a hysterectomy, although infrequently, a woman loses a significant amount of blood, making a blood transfusion necessary. Most people having major surgery today now use *autologous transfusion*, donating their own blood ahead of time for this purpose. Although the blood available in blood banks is extremely safe, the safest possible transfusion is your own blood, which can be stored in a blood bank for two to three weeks before the surgery. Then, if you do need blood, using your own prebanked blood reduces the possibility of a transfusion reaction. Since banking autologous (your own) blood is a common practice, many blood banks have specific procedures to expedite this. If you do bank your own blood, you should take an iron supplement before and after your blood is collected to enhance your body's production of new red blood cells.

A hospital blood bank will not accept autologous blood donations from a woman who is anemic. Many women who are scheduled for hysterectomy have a history of excessive vaginal bleeding—after all, bleeding is a common reason for surgery in the first place—and anemia. If your blood count (hemoglobin and hematocrit) is too low for you to provide one or two units of your own blood safely for storage, you may be given a drug (GnRH analog) that will stop the vaginal bleeding, enabling you to build up your own blood count through treatment with iron and ultimately bank your own blood.

Most hospital blood banks discourage directed donations by friends and relatives. Usually the blood type is incompatible, and therefore the blood is not usable by the patient anyway. Blood from directed donation also needs to be extensively screened, including for hepatitis and HIV as well as for compatibility.

If you cannot bank autologous blood and you need a transfusion, the hospital will provide units of blood that match your blood type. These units are screened for unusual antibodies and compatibility to your blood type and are tested to allow matching of blood type and to minimize the risk of an adverse transfusion reaction. Blood banks are required to test every unit of donated blood for infectious diseases (for example, HIV, syphilis, hepatitis).

ANESTHESIA

Anesthesiology Consultation

You may wish to talk to the anesthesiologist who will be involved with your surgery shortly before the operation. Ask your doctor to provide relevant laboratory data and other preoperative information to the anesthesiologist before the time of the assessment so that the anesthesiologist can take this information into account in his or her discussion with you.

The anesthesiologist will evaluate your anesthetic risks and discuss your preferences (for example, general or regional anesthetic). The anesthesiologist, sometimes in collaboration with the surgeon, will then determine the type of anesthesia that will be used during your surgery. The surgical approach (abdominal, vaginal, or laparoscopic) is a factor in determining anesthesia. If the laparoscopic approach is used, you will need a general anesthetic because the peritoneal cavity is filled with gas as part of the procedure for laparoscopy in order to keep the intestinal tract structures out of the way and the abdominal wall from collapsing. The presence of this gas makes expanding the lungs difficult, if not impossible, without general anesthesia and associated muscle-relaxing drugs.

Years ago, patients who were to have major surgery were admitted to the hospital for evaluation at least a day before their operation and routinely met their anesthesiologist in the hospital the day before surgery. In current hospital practice, with emphasis on shortened lengths of stay, women having hysterectomies are almost always admitted on the same day as the surgery. It is possible that you will not speak with the anesthesiologist until shortly before your hysterectomy.

We recommend a consultation before the day of surgery if possible, especially if there are any medical issues that could affect the administration of anesthesia. If you have a history of a significant medical illness or are under treatment for a medical disease, you should schedule a preoperative anesthesiology evaluation at least two working days ahead of your admission to the hospital for the surgery. Such illnesses include heart disease (coronary artery disease, valvular disease excluding mitral valve prolapse, arrhythmias), severe asthma, chronic obstructive pulmonary disease, emphysema, diabetes, thyroid disease, sleep apnea, and morbid obesity. In addition, any woman over the age of 50 should have preoperative clearance from her primary care physician or have a preoperative anesthesia evaluation. Even if you don't fit into any of these categories, if you are more comfortable with an anesthesia evaluation before you go into the hospital, you should ask for a consultation.

The American Society of Anesthesiology lists a number of different conditions under various classifications for which consultation before the day of surgery is recommended. The severity of the disorder will determine whether an anesthesiologist or a nurse practitioner conducts the consultation. The classifications and specific conditions are as follows:

- General medical condition: Any medical condition that has kept a person from engaging in normal daily activities or has required continuous assistance or monitoring at home in the six months prior to surgery; or admission to the hospital in the two months prior to surgery because of acute flare-up of a chronic condition.
- Cardiovascular: History of angina, coronary artery disease, or heart attack; arrhythmias (irregular heartbeat) that cause symptoms; poorly controlled high blood pressure; or history of congestive heart failure.
- Respiratory: Asthma or chronic obstructive pulmonary disease requiring chronic medication, or with problems or progression within six month prior to surgery; any history of major surgery on the airway or anatomic abnormalities in the airway; tumor or obstruction of the airway; history of chronic respiratory distress requiring home ventilation.
- Endocrine: Diabetes for which insulin or oral medication is needed for control; adrenal disorders; active thyroid disease.
- Neuromuscular: History of seizure disorder or other significant central nervous system disease such as multiple sclerosis, myasthenia gravis; history of muscle disorder.
- Liver: Any active liver-related disease.
- Musculoskeletal: Conditions that compromise function such as severe scoliosis; temporomandibular joint disorder; cervical or thoracic spine injury.
- Oncology: Current treatment with chemotherapy or weakened physical condition because of cancer or treatment for cancer.
- Gastrointestinal: Massive obesity (more than 140% of ideal body weight); symptomatic gastroesophageal reflux.

Types of Anesthesia

The most common types of anesthesia used for hysterectomy are general and epidural. Less frequently, spinal anesthesia is used. Epidurals are usually preferred because with a spinal the anesthetic agent cannot be reinstilled. This limits the amount of time that the anesthetic will work, and so the procedure must be done more quickly.

In general anesthesia, the anesthesiologist induces a state of unconsciousness in the patient. Either the patient inhales a drug to induce this state, or the drug is administered intravenously. General anesthesia also deadens pain and causes muscles to relax. Usually a combination of drugs is used to achieve these purposes. Although risks of general anesthesia are low, these drugs affect all areas of your body, including your heart and brain. Risks include postsurgical nausea and vomiting, sore throat, and muscle pain. More serious possibilities include stress on the heart, irregular heartbeat, and—very rarely—heart attack, stroke, brain damage, or death.

Spinals and epidurals are regional anesthetics, in which the spinal cord or large groups of nerves are blocked, numbing the area. Sometimes intravenous sedatives are given along with the regional anesthesia, so that you will be asleep or very drowsy during the operation, but this is not the same "sleep" induced by general anesthesia. One of the risks of regional anesthetics is postoperative headaches, especially from a spinal. Other risks of regional anesthesia include discomfort because the anesthetic does not sufficiently numb the area, allergic reaction to the anesthetic, nerve damage, breathing problems, and, rarely, seizures, cardiac arrest, dizziness, or loss of consciousness.

For a spinal, the anesthesiologist inserts a catheter into the space between the spinal cord and the dura mater, the tough membrane that surrounds the cord. An epidural is somewhat less invasive—the catheter is inserted into the epidural space, the area outside the dura. The tiny catheter used in an epidural may remain in place after surgery, and pain-relieving medications can be administered through the catheter. By pushing a button, a woman can control her own pain medication based on what she thinks she needs. (The device is programmed to prevent an overdose.) This form of postoperative pain relief is called *patient-controlled analgesia* (PCA). Alternatively, PCA may be administered intravenously with comparable pain relief.

The choice of anesthesia will involve a consideration of the woman's age and state of health as well as the specific surgical approach, other procedures being done during the same surgery, and anticipated time requirements of the surgery. For example, for women with asthma or other lung diseases, regional anesthesia is preferable to general anesthesia because there is less possibility of respiratory complications. For women who have a problem with blood clotting or women who are taking an anticoagulant, an epidural or spinal may not be optimal because of the risk of bleeding into the spinal canal. Again, general anesthesia is necessary for a laparoscopic operation.

THINGS YOU CAN DO TO PREPARE

Women preparing for hysterectomy (or any other surgical procedure) might feel they have handed over control of their lives to their surgeons and there is not much they can do for themselves. In fact, we suggest that our patients look at this experience as a partnership. We offer several tips that arise from the above discussion, things you can do to help yourself at this time in your life:

- If you are a smoker, it is best to avoid smoking for *at least* two weeks before your surgery to reduce the chance of a pulmonary infection and to make anesthesia easier.
- Stop taking aspirin two weeks before surgery, unless it is being used for a serious medical condition for which there is no suitable alternative.
- Make certain your gynecologist and anesthesiologist know what medications you are taking so that they can be ordered for you for after the surgery without significant interruption. Some hospitals object to patients bringing in and taking their own medications while they are hospitalized.
- If you are on daily medications, be certain to tell your doctor if you have omitted a dose while fasting in preparation for surgery. Some medications *should* be administered on the day of surgery by the anesthesiologist (for example, beta blockers, insulin, corticosteroids).
- Try to get a good night's sleep the night prior to surgery.
- Take no food or fluids by mouth after midnight prior to surgery.
- Leave valuables (jewelry, money) at home.
- Check with your doctor about whether you should take an enema or use a laxative before surgery to empty your lower intestinal tract. This cleansing of the bowel is commonly referred to as a *bowel prep*. Various methods are used for bowel prep, depending on how

clean the intestinal tract needs to be for your particular surgery. You may be asked to use an enema on the night prior to surgery in order to empty the lower bowel, or you may be asked to drink only liquids on the day before surgery and to take a gallon of Go-lytely, a solution that enhances bowel emptying, during the day for a more complete evacuation of the bowel contents. Sometimes a course of various antibiotics is prescribed to sterilize the bowel prior to surgery.

These measures may be recommended especially if your doctor thinks that the surgery will involve surgically separating the bowel from the pelvic structures. This may be the case if there are pelvic adhesions involving the bowel, or if you have extensive en-dometriosis, a large ovarian mass that may be stuck to the bowel, or if the surgery is being done to treat ovarian or endometrial can-cer. Your doctor may also routinely ask that you do a bowel prep as a precaution, in case more extensive disease than expected is found during surgery.

Cleansing the bowel will make the surgery easier to perform for your physician and will reduce the risk of widespread infection if the bowel is inadvertently injured during the surgery. In addition, a bowel prep will likely contribute to your comfort immediately after surgery, since anesthesia often slows the bowel activity. Thus, it may take several days to resume normal bowel function. A full bowel at the time of surgery may contribute to lower abdominal discomfort after surgery.

CHAPTER 10

What Happens in the Hospital

Hysterectomy involves a series of progressive steps, and the surgeon doing the operation will break it down that way. He opens the skin, ties off the blood vessels, and gets through the abdominal wall. He sutures the ligaments and vessels that connect the uterus to the rest of the pelvic structures, extracts the uterus, examines the abdominal cavity and surrounding area, and closes up the incision. We think of an expression we heard growing up: *Life is hard by the yard but a cinch by the inch.* In this chapter, we break down the hysterectomy procedure to inches, the succession of small steps that you will experience, and explain them.

Having any kind of surgery can be a formidable experience for anyone. As we have suggested, knowing what to expect is a tremendous help in easing fears and helping you feel in control. In this chapter we tell you what happens from the time you arrive at the hospital to check in for your hysterectomy to the time you are discharged.

BEING ADMITTED

Hysterectomy is almost always same-day surgery; that is, you are operated on the same day you are admitted to the hospital. You will probably be asked to arrive in the early morning, at least two hours before the scheduled time of surgery.

When you are admitted to the hospital, you will be asked for insurance information. Make sure you have your insurance card handy. You will be asked to complete forms, indicating who is responsible for fees not covered by insurance. Other forms will give consent for the surgery and will list potential complications. You will also be asked whether you have ever completed advance directive forms and, if so, where they are located. Take your time with the forms, read the fine print, and ask any questions that come to mind.

You will meet your anesthesiologist, if you have not done so previously, and find out your type of anesthesia. (See previous chapter for details about an anesthesiology consult.) Members of the nursing staff will meet you in the preoperative area. You may also meet a resident or other physician who will assist your surgeon in the operating room. A nurse will ask you questions about your health and medical history, medications you take, and any allergies you have and will check your preoperative laboratory tests and operative forms. Sometimes it might feel as if you have answered the same questions a dozen times, but try to be patient and continue to give comprehensive answers. It is for your own health that this information is being collected and recorded again.

PREOPERATIVE PROCEDURES

Now that you have met your surgical team, the procedures will begin. The first thing necessary is to make a vein easily accessible to administer medications and fluid. This is done with an intravenous needle, commonly known as an IV. When done properly, IV insertion is quick and painless. A nurse or a specialized IV technician will usually put in the IV, inserting the needle into a vein in one of your hands or arms and running intravenous fluids through a tube into the needle and vein. This will ensure that you are well hydrated and have an intravenous line for administration of medications and additional fluids during surgery. This IV line will remain in place throughout surgery and after, until you are taking fluids by mouth and no longer need intravenous medications.

Usually, a dose of an antibiotic is given through your intravenous access line before surgery to prevent infection. Be sure to tell your doctors if you are allergic to any antibiotics (or any other drugs) or if you have a heart murmur, which in itself is reason to administer specific antibiotics before surgery (to protect the heart from infection).

After these preliminaries to surgery are completed in the preoperative area of the operating suite, you will be taken to the operating room, usually walking under your own steam but possibly in a wheelchair or on a bed. This isn't entirely unfamiliar to most people—many of us have seen vivid depictions of surgery on television, including real-life documentaries of actual surgical procedures. Once you are in the operating room, you will move to an operating room table. Monitors will be placed on your chest, arms, and finger by the anesthesiologist, and a blood pressure cuff will be placed around the upper portion of your arm so that your heart rate, blood pressure, and status of oxygenation can be checked regularly.

In the Operating Room

The choice of anesthesia will already have been made, based on the type of surgical approach, your medical condition, the predicted length of the operation, and your own preferences. General anesthesia is induced by medications given directly through the intravenous tubing. Once the general anesthesia takes effect, you will be asleep. During the course of the operation, additional anesthesia agents are administered either through the intravenous line, by a face mask, or through a breathing tube (endotracheal tube), which is placed through your mouth into your windpipe. This tube is inserted while you are asleep and is removed shortly after the surgery is completed, generally before you wake up. It is unlikely that you will have any memory of breathing through a tube.

If you have regional anesthesia—either spinal or epidural (or, for some women, a combination of both)—you will not be asleep unless your anesthesiologist provides supplemental intravenous sedation, as is often done. You may prefer not to have sedation. If so, be certain to discuss your preference with the anesthesiologist. Regional anesthesia, as explained in the previous chapter, blocks the nerves to the part of your body in which the surgery is being performed. The anesthetic medication is inserted through a needle or catheter placed through the lower back to the region of your spine. This medication bathes the nerves to the pelvic area as they leave the spinal cord. Thus, there is no sensation of pain in the surgical area, and it is numb as long as the anesthetic remains in effect. Many anesthesiologists, surgeons, and patients prefer regional anesthesia because it is associated with fewer pulmonary (lung) complications after surgery.

The use of an epidural catheter to provide continuous regional anesthesia during the surgery also makes it possible for postoperative pain relief to be delivered through the catheter. As mentioned in Chapter 9, with patient-controlled analgesia (PCA) the patient can press a button to release a small amount of medication into the epidural catheter for pain relief. PCA is used for one to three days after the surgery.

Once anesthesia has been administered, the surgeon usually inserts a Foley catheter through the urethra and into the bladder to help drain the bladder so the surgeon can monitor your fluid output accurately. The urinary tract catheter also spares you the need to use a bedpan immediately after the operation. In most cases the catheter is removed on the morning following surgery; its removal involves only minimal discomfort.

Finally, the abdomen and vagina are cleaned with antiseptic solutions, and abdominal or pubic hair (or both) may be shaved. Drapes are placed to cover your entire body with the exception of the site of the incision, and the surgery begins.

SOME QUESTIONS AND ANSWERS

The details of what happens next in the operating room are covered extensively in Chapter 11, which explains the different types of hysterectomy. Here we address general questions that we commonly encounter. Although many women generally have similar questions about their surgery, the same answer does not always apply for everyone. We will provide a range of possible answers to a number of frequently asked questions.

How Long Will It Take?

The length of the procedure varies from as little as one hour to four to six hours, depending on the underlying problem, the surgical approach, the individual's anatomy, and the complexity of the operation. Most hysterectomy surgeries take about two hours.

How Will I Feel When I Wake Up?

This depends on the anesthesia and the type of procedure. If you had general anesthesia, you may feel groggy, and you may experience nausea. If you have pain, you will be given pain medication to make it tolerable. Most women who use patient-controlled analgesic, the device that allows you to administer frequent small doses of a painkiller, are very satisfied with the way it controls pain. Some women (especially if they develop a postoperative infection) may be more bothered by the pain (but rarely for more than a couple of days).

What Activities Can I Do after Surgery?

Some physicians request that women be helped into a chair on the evening of surgery to maximize circulation to the legs. You will be encouraged to walk short distances soon after the surgery, usually the next morning. How quickly you pick up your level of activity will depend on the type of surgery you had and your physical condition prior to surgery.

How Long Will I Be in the Hospital?

Some women are able to leave the hospital within twenty-four hours of their surgery, but others need more time in the hospital. This depends on the extent of surgery, the woman's age and health, and other medical conditions. Generally, women stay in the hospital for one to two days after a vaginal or laparoscope-assisted vaginal hysterectomy and two to three days after a simple abdominal hysterectomy.

After a hysterectomy, it is usually recommended that women see their doctor at three weeks and then again at six weeks following surgery. The precise time for postoperative visits will be stipulated by your doctor.

When Can I Resume All My Usual Activities?

Resumption of activities varies from woman to woman, depending on many of the factors mentioned earlier. You will increase your activities daily, beginning with short walks. Stairs may be difficult at first, especially after an abdominal incision, and should be taken with caution, one step at a time, placing both feet on each step, as young children do. Be sure to hold on to the railing. Your strength will return within one to two weeks. You will probably be able to drive after three weeks and resume all your previous activities within six weeks.

Women who take baths will probably want to switch to showers for the first couple of weeks after surgery because of difficulty getting into and out of the bathtub.

Some women recover more slowly than others. Leslie is an example of someone who took a long time to get back to normal.

🦶 *It was almost a year after her hysterectomy that Leslie finally felt she had her old energy back, that she could bounce up and down the stairs, bend down to pick something up off the floor without thinking about it. For the first couple of days after she was home from the hospital she slept a lot, and for weeks after that she was astonished at how fatigued she would become from the slightest activity. A corporate administrator, she was back at work part-time at ten days following surgery, with someone driving her to work, and full-time in six weeks. But she was very thankful she had a desk job that was not physically taxing. She gradually got her energy back but was surprised by how long it took.*

Martha recovered more quickly.

🦶 *When Martha got home from the hospital four days after her hysterectomy, she treated herself more gently than usual, setting up a bed on the first floor for herself and avoiding stairs for three weeks. A visiting nurse walked with her every day, and she slowly began an exercise program, being very careful not to overdo it.*

And Beverly felt unwell for more than a week but then quickly turned the corner.

🦶 *For nine days after her hysterectomy, Beverly felt pain at the site of her abdominal incision, along with cramping and bleeding. Then she suddenly felt better. "Bam, I just turned the corner," she recalls. "At three weeks I was ready to go back to work part-time, and my only problem since then has been weight gain."*

Will I Be Able to Resume My Normal Lifestyle?

Within six weeks almost all women who have had hysterectomies are back to their full range of presurgery daily activities, including working, driving, shopping, child care, housework, and exercising. We recommend that you add activities gradually, paying close attention to your body and the way it responds to the tasks you attempt. If you feel pain or undue fatigue, slow down and wait a little to try again. Many women who have hysterectomy soon realize that, without the limitations imposed by the conditions that pushed them to surgery, their level of activity has been enhanced. In other words, normal gets better.

How Can I Avoid Gaining Weight after Surgery?

Weight gain is a common complaint after hysterectomy, but the weight gain is probably not directly related to the procedure. During the recovery period, women are less active and may change their eating habits because they often are home rather than leading an active life. They may also be fatigued, because of blood loss or simply because of the surgical procedure. It is possible that women become less active and exercise less after the recovery period because they have gotten out of the habit, leading to weight gain. After the six-week recovery period, if eating habits and activity levels return to baseline, then weight should not change.

When Can I Resume Sexual Activity? Will I Notice Any Difference in Sexual Function?

We tell women that they will be able to resume sexual relations four to six weeks after surgery. Many women find that their sex life improves after hysterectomy, without the gynecologic problem they had been struggling with, often for years. One recent study of sexuality after hysterectomy concluded that there was no evidence that hysterectomy had any detrimental effect on sexuality—its effect was either neutral or enhancing. (See Chapter 12.)

Will My Hormone Balance Change after Surgery?

Your hormone balance almost certainly will not change unless your ovaries are removed. In rare instances, primarily associated with anatomic distortions, hysterectomy may compromise the blood supply to the ovaries, leading to a hormonal deficiency. See Chapter 13 for a complete discussion of hormone replacement therapy, recommended for some women to restore a healthful hormone balance.

What Will You Do If You Find Something Unexpected?

This, of course, depends on many factors. You should explore this question with your doctor. Ask your doctor, for example, what he would do if he found an unexpected malignancy or another condition more serious than previously expected.

What Goes in the Space My Uterus Used to Occupy?

Many women are concerned about what happens after hysterectomy to the space in their abdomen that was once occupied by the uterus and other pelvic organs that have been removed. In fact, the uterus, tubes, and ovaries take up only a small amount of the total volume of the pelvic cavity. The normal uterus is typically the size of a small pear, the ovaries are each usually about the size of an apricot, and the fallopian tubes are approximately the diameter and length of a pencil. When these structures are removed, the bowel fills the space they previously occupied. The same phenomenon occurs when the uterus shrinks in size immediately after the birth of a baby.

SURGICAL APPROACHES

The three basic surgical approaches to hysterectomy are

1. abdominal, which requires an abdominal incision;
2. vaginal, in which the uterus is removed through the vagina; and
3. laparoscope-assisted vaginal hysterectomy (LAVH), in which a laparoscope (telescope) is inserted through a tiny abdominal incision, laser or electrocautery tools are inserted through additional small incisions, and these instruments are used to free the uterus from its attachments so it can be removed through the vagina.

The details of these different approaches are provided in Chapter 11. The vaginal approach is becoming increasingly popular—over the past two decades the proportion of vaginal procedures has risen from 26 to 32 percent of all hysterectomies. Laparoscopic surgery has made the vaginal approach possible in women who would have had abdominal surgery for hysterectomy in the past. About 15 percent of vaginal hysterectomies are done with laparoscopic assistance.

Recently, some gynecologists have advocated a return to performing *supracervical hysterectomy*—removing the body of the uterus but not the cervix. This is also referred to as a *subtotal hysterectomy*. We discuss the advantages and disadvantages of preserving the cervix in Chapter 11.

Hysterectomy does *not* imply removal of the ovaries and fallopian tubes. These procedures, called oophorectomy and salpingectomy, are sometimes done along with hysterectomy, but only if there are specific reasons to do so.

POTENTIAL COMPLICATIONS OF HYSTERECTOMY

As you move through the steps of hysterectomy, you will undoubtedly give some thought to what could go wrong. A preponderance of evidence indicates that hysterectomy is generally a safe procedure, but some women will develop complications, and in very rare instances there have even been deaths. (Currently the mortality rate for hysterectomy is less than 0.1%.) Complications can be divided into two categories: problems related to the operation (during surgery) and problems in the postoperative period (after surgery).

A list of complications might look like an alarming catalogue of dire possibilities, and our purpose here is not to frighten or deter you. Most often when complications do occur, they are mild, but we believe it is helpful at least to be aware of the worst-case scenarios in order to be prepared for whatever happens. One study of more than one thousand women who had hysterectomies found that nearly 67 percent experienced mild complications such as nausea or vomiting; 11 percent had moderate complications such as failure of the incision to heal properly; and fewer than 1 percent had serious complications such as pulmonary embolism (a blood clot in an artery leading to the lungs).

The American College of Obstetricians and Gynecologists (ACOG) estimates that from 25 to 50 percent of women who have hysterectomies experience some sort of problem related to the surgery, either during surgery or in the immediate postoperative period. Fever and bleeding are most commonly reported. Some problems may not appear until weeks or even months after surgery. In an ACOG-recommended consent form for hysterectomy, the following possible complications are listed:

- Nausea
- Vomiting
- Pain
- Bleeding
- Infection
- Poor healing

- Hernia
- Formation of adhesions
- Unexpected drug reactions
- Unintended injury to pelvic or abdominal structures including fallopian tubes, ovaries, bladder, ureter, or bowel
- Nerve injury
- Blood clots

In addition, many women experience fatigue and weight gain after hysterectomy. The weight gain is related primarily to decreased activity, possibly as a result of fatigue during convalescence. It is not a consequence of hysterectomy per se. Long-term psychological effects may include depression, although more often we find that women experience a sense of well-being once hysterectomy has solved their gynecologic problems. Not surprisingly, depression is sometimes observed in women who had been unsuccessful in their attempts at conception and pregnancy and must now face the finality of their inability to give birth. (See Chapter 12 for a discussion of childbirth alternatives.)

In general, complications during LAVH are more likely to include laceration of blood vessels, nerves, or adjacent organs within the abdomen. Urinary complications occur more frequently with vaginal hysterectomy. However, it may not be valid to compare the complications of these different approaches to surgery, since vaginal hysterectomy is often selected when technical difficulties are not anticipated. In the following chapter, we discuss complications for each of the different surgical approaches used for hysterectomy.

SURGICAL MENOPAUSE ASSOCIATED WITH HYSTERECTOMY

More than half of women who undergo hysterectomy also have both of their ovaries removed at the same time. This procedure, *bilateral oophorectomy*, is being done with hysterectomy more frequently than in the past—the percentage has increased through the years, from 25 percent in 1965 to 41 percent in 1985, 47 percent in 1988, and 52 percent in 1993.

The reasons for having an oophorectomy are discussed in the next chapter. Women who are older at the time of their surgery are more likely to have their ovaries removed at the time of the hysterectomy because the closer a woman is to menopause, the less ovarian function and hormone production she has remaining. Between 1988 and 1993, more than three-quarters of women aged 45 to 54 had their ovaries removed at the time of hysterectomy. The reason for removing normal ovaries is to reduce the woman's risk of developing ovarian cancer. A woman must weigh how long the ovaries will continue to produce hormones if they are not removed against the possible development of ovarian cancer in her lifetime. The lifetime risk for a woman to develop ovarian cancer is 1–2 percent.

Oophorectomy causes menopause—referred to as *surgical menopause* because it is the result of surgery rather than of natural aging. Menopausal women who have had a hysterectomy and women who become surgically menopausal have an advantage if they decide to take hormone replacement therapy. Since they no longer have a uterus, the possibility of uterine bleeding that may occur with estrogen therapy is eliminated. Furthermore, taking a progestin along with estrogen is unnecessary because the possibility of developing endometrial (uterine) cancer no longer exists. (Hormone replacement therapy is discussed in Chapter 13.)

YOUR HOSPITAL STAY

When Martha woke up from her abdominal hysterectomy, she felt like she'd been run over by a truck. She was very thankful that she was in a hospital, with people taking care of her. During her four days at the hospital, she gradually started feeling better, but she decided that she would be very careful about resuming her normal activities when she returned home.

The hospital staff will start working with you toward your recovery from the time you awaken from anesthesia. Usually during surgery you will have a catheter in your bladder through which urine exits the body; by the morning after surgery, the catheter will be removed. That same morning, your nurse will assist you in getting out of bed and will help you walk to the bathroom. You want to be up and about as soon as possible after abdominal surgery—the longer you put it off, the more difficult or painful it will be to move around. After vaginal surgery, it will not be as difficult or painful to move around because your abdominal muscles have not been cut.

You will continue to receive fluids through the intravenous line until you are able to take them by mouth, which is usually on the first postoperative day. Often pain medicine is delivered on an "as-needed" basis via the IV or epidural catheter. Narcotics are generally prescribed for severe pain. However, narcotic medications often slow down return of bowel function, slow recovery in general, and make you feel "fuzzy." Use of nonsteroidal anti-inflammatory medications such as ibuprofen or naproxen may alleviate pain without the negative effects of narcotics.

The timing for removing stitches or staples from the incision varies depending on the surgeon's preference. Usually sutures are removed on the day of your discharge from the hospital. If not, your surgeon will probably have you return to the office within several days to a week after discharge to remove skin sutures or staples; the surgeon will examine the incision at that time. *Subcuticular stitches* are absorbable stitches placed in the tissue just beneath the skin. They dissolve over several weeks and never require removal.

In the hospital, and later, when you are at home recovering, certain signs and symptoms could indicate serious complications. Alert your nurse or doctor in the hospital if you feel dizzy, nauseated, or short of breath or if you experience significant pain. In the hospital, your vital signs will be taken regularly to monitor for fever or changes in blood pressure, and your bleeding and urine output also will be monitored.

GOING HOME

 Kristine was so delighted that her hysterectomy relieved her many symptoms from fibroids that she tried to resume some of her previous activities a bit too quickly. She waited six weeks to go back to work, as her surgeon had advised. But her job as a medical researcher required that she be on her feet a great deal, and after only half a day Kristine knew she wasn't ready for it. She worked a couple of half days and was much more tired than she'd expected. Her boss was sympathetic when she told him she needed more time off, and she stayed home for another week. When she returned to work the second time, she felt much stronger and had no trouble working full days and doing her job.

Getting back to normal is different for every woman—just as different women heal differently and have different demands in their daily lives.

We have presented guidelines for resuming activities in the question-and-answer section above. What is most important is for every woman to know the symptoms of a problem and catch it early. With today's shorter hospitalizations, a woman is more responsible than ever before to monitor her own well-being.

Occasionally, postoperative problems develop at home. Most of the time these are not serious. Once you are home from the hospital, call your doctor if you have any of the following symptoms; if you can't quickly reach your doctor and feel your problem is serious, go to an emergency room:

- Fever, which is usually a sign of infection. When a woman goes home after only a brief hospitalization, infection may show up after she is home.
- Dizziness or feeling faint
- Nausea and vomiting
- Shortness of breath
- Significant (heavy, prolonged) bleeding from the vagina
- Leakage from the incision, or the incision site opens up
- Pain when urinating
- Involuntary loss of urine
- Abdominal, leg, or chest pain
- Swelling or redness in a leg

For the most part, recovery from a hysterectomy is straightforward and uneventful.

Within a couple of months of her hysterectomy, Helena felt "great," with more energy than she'd had for years. No longer dragging through the days, no more bleeding, no more scheduling her life around her monthly cycles. She felt like a new person with a new life.

CHAPTER 11

What Kind of Hysterectomy Should You Have?

I f you are going to have a hysterectomy, you will want to know which surgical approach will be used: abdominal, vaginal, or laparoscopic. You will also want to know which organs and how much surrounding tissue will be removed (the *extent* of surgery). The decision about surgical approach and the decision about extent of surgery are often interrelated and are usually made together. The extent of surgery determines whether the hysterectomy is referred to as *total* or *subtotal, simple* or *radical.*

- When the uterus is removed in its entirety along with the cervix, the procedure is a *total* hysterectomy.
- When the uterus is removed but the cervix is not, the procedure is called a *subtotal* or *supracervical* hysterectomy.
- A *simple* hysterectomy is removal of the uterus without removal of adjacent tissue or lymph nodes. It can be abdominal, vaginal, or laparoscopic.
- A *radical* hysterectomy involves removal of the uterus but also the upper third of the vagina (including the cervix), tissue immediately adjacent to the uterus, and pelvic lymph nodes. This procedure is usually done to treat cancer, especially cervical cancer.

In this chapter we describe these different types of hysterectomy and then the surgical approaches to hysterectomy. At the end of the chapter we describe cesarean hysterectomy, a procedure that is rarely done today.

TYPES OF HYSTERECTOMY
Total or Subtotal?

℀ For four years, Christa's fibroids had been a problem. As the months went by, the pain in her abdomen and the bleeding got worse, and then she developed anemia and weakness because of the bleeding. The pain was not incapacitating, but every time she moved, she felt tugging sensations in her abdomen. She was ready for a hysterectomy. She was 52 years old with nearly grown children, and she didn't want to be bothered with gynecologic concerns anymore. She wanted her uterus, cervix, and ovaries removed—in addition to getting relief from her current problems, she didn't want ever to have to worry about getting cancer in any of these organs.

When an abdominal hysterectomy is performed and the cervix is removed, that is a total hysterectomy. There has been a trend recently toward the supracervical (or subtotal) hysterectomy—removing the body of the uterus but not the cervix. A subtotal hysterectomy is a simpler procedure than a total hysterectomy. It takes less operating time, can be performed through a smaller abdominal incision, and is usually associated with fewer complications during surgery and fewer postoperative complications such as vaginal prolapse. However, we recommend caution in choosing this approach because it still leaves a woman at risk of contracting cervical cancer.

Removal of the cervix during hysterectomy is somewhat controversial. Some doctors believe that the cervix plays an important role in sexual responsiveness. We do not believe the cervix has a significant function when the uterus is absent, but there have been limited anecdotal reports (though not yet substantiated by scientific study) suggesting that the cervix has a role in sexual stimulation during intercourse. Women who have undergone total hysterectomy continue to experience orgasm and continue to provide their own lubrication of the vaginal walls, unless they lacking adequate estrogen.

Supracervical hysterectomy was preferred in years past because it was easier to perform and carried with it half the mortality rate of total hysterectomy. It also left a woman at risk for cervical cancer. In the decades preceding Pap smears, most surgeons took advantage of better anesthesia and the availability of blood transfusion and antibiotics and chose to perform a total hysterectomy, removing the cervix as well as the uterine body in order to prevent cervical cancer.

Surgical practice has again changed with the advent of reliable Pap testing and thus a greater chance of detecting very early cervical cancer, the ability (through HPV testing) to identify women at high risk for cervical cancer, and the very small risks (1 per 1,000) of cancer developing in the cervical stump that may remain. Supracervical hysterectomy is an acceptable choice for some women today.

Conserving the cervix protects the cardinal ligaments, which provide support for the vagina, and reduces vaginal prolapse. However, appropriate attention to correct suturing of these ligaments after removal of the cervix should provide ample support for the top of the vagina. (See Chapter 1.) In most women, we have not seen evidence to support the idea that supracervical has great advantages over total hysterectomy.

Women who have supracervical hysterectomies must remember that they need to continue to have regular Pap tests. Retaining the cervix is an option only when the cervix is normal and Pap smears have never revealed any significant or suspicious abnormalities—in other words, only in women at low risk for developing cervical cancer. If your hysterectomy is being performed for a reproductive tract malignancy or premalignant disease, you should *not* have your cervix conserved.

There are some other reasons to remove the cervix together with the uterus. If the cervix is removed, you don't need to have annual Pap smears because you have virtually no possibility of getting cervical cancer. In addition, menstrual periods will occasionally occur after subtotal hysterectomy, when a portion of the lower segment of the uterus is left attached to the spared cervix. If the cervix is retained, bleeding can also occur from trauma, infection, or development of a cervical polyp. Under these circumstances, careful investigation is necessary to exclude the possibility of cervical cancer. If you have a hysterectomy for endometriosis or a chronic pelvic infection, retaining the cervix may enable endometriosis to recur within the cervical tissue.

If your hysterectomy is performed for a benign condition, you should ask your physician her opinions about cervical removal. If you are at low risk for developing cervical cancer and wish to have a supracervical hysterectomy because of worry over your future sexuality if the cervix is removed, or because of other concerns, your doctor should honor your wishes. But it is important that you realize and appreciate the potential risks detailed here (for example, the potential for cervical problems, including cancer).

Simple and Radical Hysterectomies

A simple hysterectomy (removal of just the uterus) can be done abdominally, vaginally, or laparoscopically. The term is used primarily to differentiate it from a radical hysterectomy, a more extensive procedure that involves removal of the uterus, the upper third of the vagina, tissue immediately adjacent to the uterus, and pelvic lymph nodes.

Radical hysterectomy was introduced in the United States in the mid-1940s and rapidly developed as an alternative to radiation therapy for treating all but the least invasive forms of cervical cancer. It has become the primary treatment for cervical cancer. The goal is to remove as much tissue as possible adjacent to the uterus, where there is potential for spread of the malignancy. The operation is much more extensive than a simple hysterectomy and carries with it the potential for serious complications because the tissue that is removed is closely linked to vital organs such as portions of the intestinal tract, the urinary bladder, and the ureters (the tubes that carry urine from the kidneys to the bladder). Injuries to the bladder and ureters are among the most common complications of the radical hysterectomy.

If you need a radical hysterectomy, it should be performed by an experienced gynecologic oncologist, a gynecologist who has been specially trained to treat cancers of the female reproductive organs. Avoiding injury to adjacent organs is key to a successful outcome from a radical hysterectomy.

A variation is the *modified radical hysterectomy*, also called an *extrafascial hysterectomy*. This procedure is done in some women with early cervical cancer such as microinvasive cancer, which has only superficially invaded the underlying tissue. In this procedure, which has a lower complication rate than the more extensive radical hysterectomy, the surgeon ensures removal of the entire cervix by cutting only the tissue around it and not cutting into the cervix itself. Ureters and their blood supply are carefully identified to reduce the possibility of injury.

It is very unusual for cervical cancer to spread to the ovaries, and it is seldom necessary to remove the ovaries during surgery for cervical cancer. This is one reason that radical hysterectomy is a better choice of therapy for cervical cancer than radiation, particularly for young women, whose ovaries are still producing hormones. Radiation usually causes the ovaries to atrophy, and they will then no longer be able to produce estrogen.

What About the Ovaries?

Hysterectomy—total or subtotal, simple or radical, abdominal or vaginal—refers only to removal of the uterus. It does *not* mean removal of the ovaries.

In fact, only rarely is it essential to remove the ovaries (and fallopian tubes) at the time of a simple hysterectomy. Again, surgical removal of the ovaries is called *oophorectomy,* and removal of the tubes is called *salpingectomy.* (*Oophor* is the technical term for anything referring to the ovaries, and *salpinx* is the technical term for the tubes.)

- *Bilateral salpingo-oophorectomy* is the removal of both tubes and both ovaries.
- *Unilateral salpingo-oophorectomy* is the removal of one tube and the ovary on the same side.
- *Unilateral oophorectomy* is the removal of one ovary.
- *Bilateral oophorectomy* is the removal of both ovaries.

Usually if an ovary is removed at the time of hysterectomy, the adjacent tube is also removed. There is no function for the tube in the absence of a uterus, and it is usually technically safer and simpler to remove the tube together with the uterus and ovary.

The decision about whether your ovaries should be removed at the time of hysterectomy will be based on your age, the condition of your ovaries, and your personal preferences. The main reason for removing the ovaries is to prevent ovarian cancer. If you have a strong family history of ovarian cancer, you may choose to have your ovaries removed, especially if you are already postmenopausal. Removal of the ovaries may also be advisable at the time of the hysterectomy if you have endometriosis.

On the other hand, if you have not gone through menopause, you may wish to maintain your ovaries because they produce the hormones estrogen, progesterone, and androgen, which are important for your overall health. The ovaries continue to produce hormones until the time of menopause, even after the uterus is removed. Obviously, if you have had a hysterectomy and no longer have a uterus, you won't continue to menstruate, but if your ovaries are intact, you will continue to experience monthly hormonal cycles, and the hormones produced will continue their preventive effects against osteoporosis and other conditions; you simply will not experience monthly bleeding. Although hormone replacement offers many benefits (see Chapter 13), it cannot do the same job as naturally produced hormones.

In premenopausal women, the current trend in surgery is not to remove the ovaries unless the woman has endometriosis or a history of recurrent ovarian cysts or pelvic inflammatory disease (PID). (PID can progress to involve the ovaries.) Women who feel strongly that they *don't* want to begin hormone replacement therapy may want to retain their ovaries, if possible, but we emphasize that if the ovaries are diseased, they should be removed.

SURGICAL APPROACHES

In table 11.1, the possible approaches to surgery are listed for many of the gynecologic problems we discussed in Part II. There are no hard-and-fast rules about the best approach for these problems, but some approaches are used more often than others for specific problems.

In this section we pick up where Chapter 10 left off, just as surgery was about to begin. We start with abdominal hysterectomy, which is the most commonly performed hysterectomy procedure, as the table indicates.

Abdominal Hysterectomy

❦ *Leslie, in her own words, "freaked out" when her doctor told her it was time for her to have a hysterectomy. Her doctor had been monitoring Leslie's fibroids for seven years, and as Leslie went through menopause, she expected them to shrink. She never had any symptoms, but even after menopause, the fibroids continued growing, and her doctor told her they would soon interfere with the functioning of some of her organs.*

Leslie was 56 and had never had surgery in her life. She was terrified of being in the hospital, afraid of anesthesia, fearful of giving up control. She felt better after her doctor went over the procedure step by step with her and

TABLE 11.1. REASONS FOR HYSTERECTOMY AND TYPES OF
PROCEDURES

Disorder	Vaginal	Laparoscope-Assisted Vaginal	Abdominal
Uterine fibroids	Occasionally	Occasionally	Usually
Pelvic inflammatory disease	Rarely	Occasionally	Usually
Recurrent dysfunctional uterine bleeding	Usually	Occasionally	Occasionally
Endometriosis	Rarely	Occasionally	Usually
Adenomyosis	Usually	Occasionally	Occasionally
Pelvic relaxation/ prolapse	Usually	Occasionally	Occasionally
Pelvic pain	Rarely	Occasionally	Usually
Cervical cancer, stage 0	Usually	Rarely	Occasionally
Cervical cancer, Stage IA, IB, IIA	Occasionally	Rarely	Usually
Endometrial cancer	Occasionally	Occasionally	Usually

Source: Adapted from C. K. Miyazawa, "Abdominal Hysterectomy," in *Gynecologic and Obstetric Surgery*, ed. D. H. Nichols (St. Louis: Mosby–Year Book, 1993), chap. 31.

her husband. She did a great deal of reading on her own and was uncom-
fortable with the antihysterectomy tone she encountered in books and In-
ternet articles on the subject. The doctor gave her the phone numbers of other
women who had had the same procedures and who were willing to discuss
their experiences with others. These connections were helpful. She did trust
her doctor, set a date for surgery, and felt a calm descend over her as the day
approached. She had an epidural anesthesia and remained awake, which re-
lieved many of her fears about anesthesia. She chose to keep her cervix but
not her ovaries and tubes. She was surprised at how quickly things moved
in the operating room. Before she knew it, the doctor was telling her that all
was fine, and he was putting in the final stitches.

An abdominal approach for hysterectomy is most frequently used for

- fibroids;
- chronic pelvic inflammatory infection or pelvic adhesions;

- endometriosis;
- cervical cancer;
- uterine cancer; and
- ovarian tumors when removal of the uterus is also advisable.

A vaginal hysterectomy may also be used to treat some of these conditions, depending on the extent of the problem and size of the uterus (see
below).

Other reasons for choosing an abdominal hysterectomy over a vaginal hysterectomy include a history of previous pelvic surgery such as
cesarean section, myomectomy, or endometriosis; having large pelvic
masses such as fibroids or ovarian cysts; and being a virgin or never having had a vaginal birth. Under most circumstances, abdominal hysterectomy is the best treatment for gynecologic cancers requiring hysterectomy. The major exception to this general principle is preinvasive
cancer of the cervix (carcinoma in situ), which is best treated with vaginal hysterectomy.

An abdominal hysterectomy is performed using an incision through
the abdominal wall (fig. 11.1). The incision can be made vertically, either
down the middle of the abdomen beginning at the navel (a *midline incision*) or to one side of the midline starting at the level of the pubic bone
and extending toward or around the navel (a *paramedian incision*). Or
the incision can be made horizontally at about the level of the pubic
hairline, the so-called bikini cut, which allows a woman to wear a bikini
without a visible scar. The horizontal approach is also referred to as a
transverse incision.

A horizontal incision provides a better cosmetic result than a vertical
one but is not advisable or feasible for all women. A vertical incision
might be preferred because of very large fibroids or extensive endometriosis, both of which require greater exposure of the organs than
a horizontal incision allows, or for cancer, when the surgeon wants to do
a complete visual assessment of the abdominal cavity to determine
whether the malignancy has spread.

In abdominal hysterectomy, the incision is made through the several layers of the abdominal wall—the skin, fat, fascia, muscle. The
uterus is separated from the ligaments and other tissue to which it is attached in the pelvis, step by step. The blood vessels supplying the uterus
are clamped and cut sequentially, and once all the attachments and blood

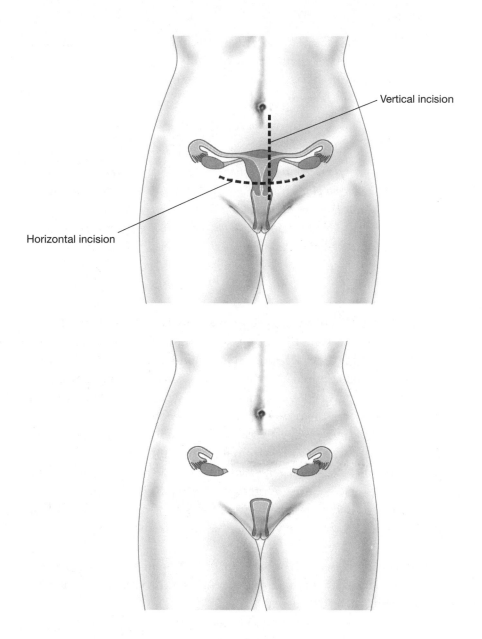

Vertical incision

Horizontal incision

FIG. 11.1. *Top:* Location of horizontal and vertical incisions used in abdominal hysterectomy. One of these incisions will be made before an abdominal hysterectomy procedure. *Bottom:* After the procedure the ovaries remain but the uterus and cervix have been removed.

vessels have been separated from the uterus, the uterus is removed from the pelvic cavity. After the surgeon carefully inspects the cavity, each of the layers is sutured back together, one by one.

Vaginal Hysterectomy

❦ Jennifer endured heavy monthly bleeding for years and started thinking about having a hysterectomy when she became so anemic that her doctor suggested she receive a blood transfusion. When she made her decision to go ahead, she wanted to have the least invasive procedure possible, and her doctor told her she was a good candidate for the vaginal approach. She was 51 when she had a vaginal hysterectomy with epidural anesthesia and came out of the surgery, in her words, "easily, with no problems." Her recovery was quick and straightforward, and she didn't look back.

One way to think of a vaginal hysterectomy is that it involves the removal of the uterus from the bottom up. In other words, the steps in the operation are done in reverse order. No abdominal incision is necessary. The only incision required is in the vaginal wall around the cervix, providing an opening big enough to remove the uterus through it. It is not possible to preserve the cervix with a vaginal approach, and so a vaginal hysterectomy is always a total hysterectomy. We always inform women who are scheduled for vaginal hysterectomy that there is a remote chance that we may have to switch to an abdominal procedure if we encounter a problem during surgery. This rarely is necessary, however.

A vaginal procedure is usually done for simpler cases. Disorders that are most frequently treated with vaginal hysterectomy are

- uterine prolapse, with or without relaxation of the vaginal walls;
- carcinoma in situ of the cervix (preinvasive cervical cancer), if hysterectomy is to be done at all;
- abnormal vaginal bleeding that doesn't respond to treatment with hormones, if a uterine malignancy has been ruled out; and
- uterine fibroids, when they have not made the uterus too large to fit through the vaginal canal.

Vaginal hysterectomy is usually *not* the best surgical approach if there is significant pelvic pathology, such as adhesions from infections or previous pelvic surgery, large pelvic masses (ovarian tumors and large uterine fibroids), or endometriosis. Women who have never had a vaginal birth are usually not able to have a vaginal hysterectomy.

Vaginal hysterectomy is frequently the approach used when a woman's uterus has prolapsed (dropped). In this condition (described in Chapter 5), the weakened tissue under the vagina may not provide sufficient support for the bladder, small bowel, and rectum, and so the surgeon repairs the pelvic floor tissues at the time of the vaginal hysterectomy. The repair procedure is called *colporrhaphy*, which means "suturing vaginal tissue"—*anterior colporrhaphy* if it is in the front, *posterior colporrhaphy* if in the back. Anterior colporrhaphy, also referred to as a *cystocele repair*, means tightening the tissue that supports the bladder. Posterior colporrhaphy (*rectocele repair*) is a similar repair of the tissue surrounding the rectum. One final term—*enterocele repair*—refers to the suturing of ligaments at the top of the vagina to prevent a portion of small intestine from pushing against the vaginal wall and eventually being eased into the vaginal canal.

Radical hysterectomy can be performed by the vaginal approach, combined with removal of lymph nodes. A radical vaginal hysterectomy is best for women who are markedly overweight, as obesity can make abdominal surgery extremely difficult.

Vaginal hysterectomy is usually a relatively simple procedure that requires less time to complete than an abdominal hysterectomy (fig. 11.2). This is because it is not necessary to make an incision that extends through the several layers of the abdominal wall, each of which needs to be sutured together individually at the conclusion of the operation. Once the anesthesia has been administered, the vaginal hysterectomy begins with the insertion of a speculum into the vagina. The surgeon makes an incision around the cervix and then clamps and cuts the supporting ligaments and the uterine artery; this process frees the uterus, which is then drawn through the incision and out of the vagina. Careful suturing of the supporting ligaments fixes them in a position to maintain support for the vagina. Ovaries and fallopian tubes can be also be removed vaginally at the time of a vaginal hysterectomy, when necessary. After surgery the opening at the top of the vagina can be closed with sutures, or it may be left open—it will seal itself closed. Leaving it open allows for drainage and poses less risk of infection.

The hospital stay after a vaginal procedure is shorter than for an ab-

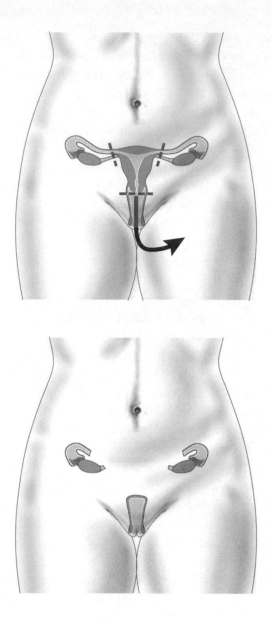

F<small>IG</small>. 11.2. Vaginal hysterectomy. *Top:* The uterus and cervix are removed through an incision in the top of the vagina. *Bottom:* After the procedure, the ovaries remain, but the uterus and cervix have been removed. Notice that the result is identical to that following abdominal hysterectomy (fig. 11.1).

dominal hysterectomy—usually either an overnight stay or, at most, one to two days. A shortened stay is possible because there are no sutures to remove and because there is less pain and discomfort after vaginal surgery than after abdominal surgery. The cosmetic benefit, of course, is that there will be no abdominal scar.

In recent years, gynecologists have favored abdominal hysterectomy over vaginal hysterectomy, in part because most contemporary medical training focuses on this approach. Nonetheless, there are many advantages to the vaginal approach—fewer complications, a shorter hospital stay, and an easier convalescence than with abdominal hysterectomy. In some studies, the overall complication rate, both major and minor, for vaginal hysterectomy has been reported at just over half that reported for abdominal hysterectomy.

Because of these advantages, gynecologic surgeons have sought improvements for the vaginal approach that could make it possible for more surgeries to be done this way. One of the areas of greatest interest has been the use of laparoscopy combined with vaginal hysterectomy.

Laparoscopic Hysterectomy

Laparoscopy is done using a lighted telescope for viewing and additional surgical instruments for cutting. All these instruments are passed into the abdominal cavity through relatively small incisions in the abdominal wall. The technique has been known for decades, but the miniaturization of equipment has expanded its role and its possibilities. Most frequently, laparoscopy is used to assist with a vaginal hysterectomy (*laparoscope-assisted vaginal hysterectomy,* or LAVH), but hysterectomy can also be done in entirety through a laparoscopic procedure (*laparoscopic hysterectomy,* or LH).

Surgeons began using laparoscopy to assist in vaginal hysterectomy in the late 1980s. In performing laparoscope-assisted vaginal hysterectomy, your doctor can combine the advantages of vaginal hysterectomy with the enhanced visualization of the pelvic organs that the laparoscope provides. LAVH is done today to treat many conditions that would have required an abdominal hysterectomy in the past, including uterine fibroids and endometriosis.

LAVH does not replace vaginal hysterectomy. Vaginal hysterectomies are still common and preferred whenever possible because they have the advantage of requiring no abdominal incision at all. LAVH is best suited for conditions in which the surgeon's ability to perform a total vaginal hysterectomy is made difficult by certain disorders (for example, endometriosis, tubal infection, or tubo-ovarian abscess) or because the woman has not given birth vaginally.

There are a number of variations in how the laparoscope is used to assist vaginal hysterectomy. They are classified into four types:

- Type 1—A laparoscope is placed to evaluate the condition of the pelvic organs and to determine whether vaginal hysterectomy is possible. In this case, the laparoscope is used only for visualization and diagnosis.
- Type 2—The laparoscope finds pelvic pathology such as adhesions or endometriosis. Your surgeon will treat these conditions through the laparoscopic incisions and then perform a vaginal hysterectomy.
- Type 3—Your doctor does part of the hysterectomy procedure through the laparoscope, a procedure called *operative laparoscopy*. For example, ligaments are cut or the blood supply to the uterus is sutured through the laparoscopic incisions. The vaginal hysterectomy is thus facilitated by the laparoscope.
- Type 4—The entire hysterectomy is performed using operative laparoscopy. The uterus is removed through the vagina, but the vaginal incision is sutured from above using the laparoscopic ports (small incisions) in the abdomen and laparoscopic instruments.

The first three options differ significantly from the fourth. They truly qualify as vaginal hysterectomy with laparoscopic *assistance* (LAVH), whereas type 4 is a complete laparoscopic hysterectomy (LH). In another variation, the surgeon uses a process called *morcellation*, which means "to divide into small pieces and remove." With laparoscopic instruments the uterus is surgically divided into small fragments, and these pieces are removed through the laparoscopic incisions. This approach requires no vaginal incision at all. However, because the bowel or other vital tissues can inadvertently be injured during morcellation, do not consider having this procedure done except by a surgeon who is very experienced with it.

Possible complications from the LAVH procedure include bleeding and injury to other organs. Since the laparoscopic instruments must be inserted through multiple small incisions into the abdominal wall (fig. 11.3), bleeding from the epigastric artery, one of the major blood vessels in the abdominal wall, can occur. Another potential complication is infection from the incision that is placed just below the navel. The medical term for this infection is *cellulitis*. More serious possible complications involve injuries to the bladder, ureters, or intestinal tract by the sharp instruments, electrocautery, or suturing techniques. Complication rates appear to be lower for LAVH than for abdominal hysterectomy but comparable for LAVH and vaginal hysterectomy.

Laparoscopic surgery has distinct advantages over an abdominal approach. It involves minimal manipulation of the intestinal tract, and bowel function usually returns promptly after surgery. The laparoscopic approach also decreases the formation of adhesions within the abdomen. Following laparoscopy, the woman is usually discharged earlier than with an abdominal hysterectomy. The recuperative phase at home is shortened, allowing a woman to resume her customary activities within two weeks.

LAVH or LH may cost more than other types of both vaginal and abdominal hysterectomy because of the expense of the specialized instruments and equipment used (many of which cannot be reused) and the longer anesthesia time. Although you will have a shorter hospital stay with LAVH, the actual surgical procedure takes longer than a vaginal hysterectomy that is not done with laparoscopic assistance. The more skilled and experienced your surgeon, the shorter the duration of the operation.

Cesarean Hysterectomy

When a hysterectomy is performed at the time of cesarean delivery of a newborn, it is often a lifesaving procedure. The need for cesarean hysterectomy is rare, occurring in one in five hundred deliveries, or one in a hundred cesarean sections, usually because of excessive uncontrolled bleeding at the time of delivery. Uncontrolled bleeding at the time of delivery most often occurs in conjunction with an abnormal placental attachment, whereby the placenta has invaded into the uterine muscle and cannot be separated without hemorrhage. This rare condition is called *placenta accreta*.

Hysterectomy may also be needed to control blood loss in the situa-

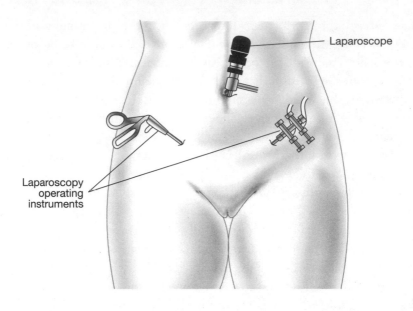

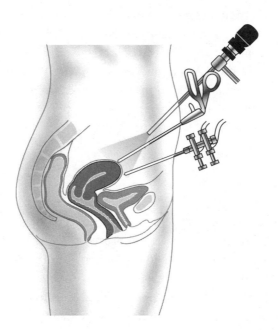

F𝗂𝗀. 11.3. Laparascopic hysterectomy showing where instruments are inserted. The laparoscope is used to visualize the structures; the laparoscopic instruments include grasping forceps, scissors, cautery, and suture holders. Three or four small abdominal incisions are made to insert the laparoscope and the laparoscopic instruments.

tion of uterine rupture, *uterine atony* (a condition in which the uterine muscle does not contract properly after delivery), or other complications of delivery resulting in extensive blood loss that cannot be controlled by other means. A hysterectomy may also be electively done at the time of cesarean section for treatment of cervical carcinoma in situ, but we do not recommend this because of the increased blood loss that is typically associated with this procedure. Blood loss is greater when a hysterectomy is done on a recently pregnant uterus because the blood vessels are larger and bleed more profusely, and it is easier to damage the urinary tract by injuring the ureters or bladder.

Although cesarean hysterectomy may have been done in the past on an elective basis for women who desired sterilization, to treat uterine fibroids, and to treat cervical carcinoma in situ, rarely is this procedure performed electively today because of the increased risk of complications.

Part IV

AFTER HYSTERECTOMY

Most women who have had hysterectomies tell us that once their hysterectomy is behind them, they can move on with their lives with an energy and focus they did not have during their years of gynecologic difficulties. Our patients have told us:

I surprised myself with how much energy I had after my recovery from the operation. I actually had a life after dinner!

Hysterectomy was a big deal because of the finality, but now that the fibroids are gone, I've never felt better. I feel extremely lucky.

If hysterectomy is medically indicated, in the long run you'll be much better off getting it done. I know that was true for me.

I do things, I go places. . . . Having a hysterectomy was the last thing I wanted, but it has turned my life around in a very positive way.

If you have had a hysterectomy, we hope that you, too, feel better and have more energy. If you are considering having a hysterectomy, you may want to talk to women who have had the surgery and can tell you about the experience and how it has affected their lives. Generally, the positives far outweigh the negatives. Nevertheless, after hysterectomy, most women also need to address a few issues, such as sexuality, hormone replacement therapy, and, for younger women, the reproductive alternatives of adoption and surrogacy. We discuss these issues in the final two chapters of our book. As always, we encourage all women to discuss their concerns with their doctor.

CHAPTER 12

Sexual and Reproductive Issues

SEX AND SEXUALITY

Many women are concerned about how hysterectomy will affect their sexuality and their sex lives. Few women feel comfortable talking with their physician about sexual matters, however, and so these concerns often remain unspoken. We urge women to become informed about this important subject before having surgery. Talk to your doctor, read books, and scout out reliable Internet sites. As we have emphasized throughout this book, women who undergo surgery fully informed tend to be more relaxed and to have better outcomes. Obtaining information about sexual response and sexual feelings is certainly no exception.

Whether your hysterectomy was done vaginally or abdominally, the surgical sites should be healed enough by about six weeks after surgery for you to have sexual intercourse without risk of infection. Before then, it's best to achieve sexual intimacy without vaginal penetration. Once you start having sexual intercourse again, if you have had your ovaries removed at the time of hysterectomy, you may discover that vaginal lubrication is a new problem, especially if you are not taking hormone replacement therapy (see the section "Lubrication" later in this chapter).

A woman's sexual desire depends on both psychological and physiological components. Physiologically, testosterone is a key hormone that influences sexual drive, and the amount of circulating testosterone affects sexual responses. Both the ovaries and the adrenal glands produce testosterone. The ovaries produce about half of all the testosterone made in a woman's body. Removal of the ovaries, therefore, lowers a woman's total testosterone level and can lead to alterations in sexual drive for some women. Even when the ovaries are not removed, the surgical procedure involved in removing the uterus may sometimes cause changes in the blood flow to the ovaries, which can lead to reduced hormonal production, including decreases in testosterone production. So even women who still have their ovaries may notice a difference in their sexual desire.

Another way pelvic surgery can adversely affect sexual desire is by making you afraid that intercourse will hurt or will injure you in some way. Your partner may have similar thoughts and may be reluctant to resume sexual intercourse for fear of injuring you internally by vaginal penetration. Once the vaginal and abdominal surgical incisions have healed, however, intercourse poses no possibility of injury.

On the other hand, the uterine disorder that prompted hysterectomy may have interfered with your normal sexual relations. Many women tell us that their sexual relations improve after hysterectomy. Hysterectomy often relieves pelvic pain or discomfort or pressure, and sexual experiences after surgery are often less inhibited and more satisfying and pleasurable.

Sexual Difficulties

🍃 *Marisol found that she didn't feel any less feminine after her hysterectomy. In fact, the opposite was true, and she felt better about her whole body than she had for some time. Her sex life continued to be a very positive part of her life.*

🍃 *For years, as Tina tried to conceive but couldn't because of severe endometriosis, she and her husband based their sexual activity on the calendar and her body temperature and not much on spontaneous desire. After her hysterectomy, when she considered her sex life, she knew that the benefits of hysterectomy far outweighed any small problems she had.*

🍃 *Sex definitely got better for Kristine after her hysterectomy. For years she had had large fibroids that caused pressure, bleeding, and pain during intercourse. After surgery, she was much more relaxed about sex than she had been before the surgery, and that new attitude translated to a much improved sex life for her and her husband.*

If you continue to have trouble with sex, don't simply accept it, thinking that's just the way it has to be. There are many ways to improve your sexual relationship and many specialists who can help you address your problems and concerns.

Lubrication. The ovaries are the main source of estrogen, a key hormone in the process of vaginal lubrication. When the ovaries are removed in conjunction with hysterectomy, estrogen levels fall rapidly. This decrease in estrogen causes vaginal dryness and painful intercourse. Hormone replacement with estrogen usually corrects this problem. In addition to oral hormone replacement therapy, estrogen can be taken through a patch or vaginally, as a cream (for example, conjugated estrogen, or estradiol cream) or an estrogen-containing tablet or ring. Note that if you have had a total hysterectomy and bilateral oophorectomy to treat a pelvic malignancy, you may not be a candidate for hormone replacement. (See Chapter 13.)

Topical vaginal lubricants that are available over the counter also are very effective at replacing natural lubrication. Astroglide, K-Y lubricant, or the contents of a vitamin E capsule can be applied vaginally to improve lubrication before intercourse.

Sexual desire. Hormone insufficiency can affect not only the physiology of sex but the psychology as well—sexual desire or libido. Adequate hormone replacement with estrogen is often all that is needed. If estrogen alone does not improve your libido, then your doctor may prescribe a combination of estrogen and an androgen such as testosterone. There is one combination medication, called Estratest, that is approved for this specific use. Or, with your doctor's instructions, a compounding pharmacist can make up a combination of estrogen and testosterone in capsule form for you to take orally or as a vaginal suppository. Soon testosterone-containing patches may be approved to increase libido in postmenopausal women.

If taking replacement hormones is not an option for you, or if these measures do not help to increase sexual desire, then take a close look at your relationship and stresses in your life for clues about changes you can make that may result in your being more receptive and relaxed. If you are working too hard or your life is stressful, try to find ways to reduce the stresses. Sometimes it is easier to blame your surgery as the cause of a sexual problem than to look further for underlying causes. A consultation with a counselor or psychologist may be helpful in providing insight into other issues in your life affecting your sexual functioning.

REPRODUCTIVE OPTIONS

Often, although hysterectomy is the best treatment available to alleviate many gynecologic conditions, it can be deferred when a woman wishes to bear children. Clearly, if hysterectomy is performed as treatment for a gynecologic malignancy, waiting is not an option. When pelvic pain from endometriosis persists despite previous conservative surgeries, when abnormal bleeding continues even though medical treatments have been tried, when the alternative treatments to hysterectomy are not well tolerated, or when a woman is simply worn down by her gynecologic problem, she may want the definitive treatment of hysterectomy.

Having children may still be an option even after hysterectomy. Adoption is the best-known alternative for couples who are unable to have children but want to have a family. A discussion of adoption is beyond our purview here, but it is a fully satisfactory way to have a family for many, many people.

Others may benefit from new reproductive technologies, which are detailed below. Since these methods involve a surrogate—another woman carrying and giving birth to a child that will be yours—it is critically important to have a legal agreement drawn up before the treatment begins. If you are investigating this method of having a child, get legal advice in the earliest stages of your considerations and remain in consultation with your lawyer throughout the process. Because of the emotional issues that surround childbirth and children, many couples exploring reproductive options also benefit from psychological counseling.

Gestational Carrier

Even if your uterus has been removed, if you have not gone through menopause and if your ovaries were not removed, then you will continue to ovulate but will no longer menstruate. Your ovaries are still producing eggs, and these eggs potentially could be used to create an embryo, if they can be collected. Today, egg collection and creation of an embryo are possible because of the many advances that have been made in the field of *in vitro fertilization* (IVF).

A woman who has had a hysterectomy but still produces eggs can have her eggs removed and fertilized with her partner's sperm. The egg or eggs are then placed in the uterus of another woman, who is known as a *gestational carrier* or *gestational surrogate* or *host uterus*. Infertile couples who attempt IVF, the so-called test-tube-baby procedure, begin by having the woman take hormones that stimulate the ovaries to produce eggs. Follicle-stimulating hormones (FSH) can be prescribed along with other medications for a woman after hysterectomy to help develop several ovarian follicles in a synchronized and coordinated fashion.

These follicles are then monitored using transvaginal ultrasound to visualize the ovaries and hormonal blood tests to ensure that the ovaries are responding to the medication appropriately. When the follicles enlarge to about 18 mm (¾ of an inch) in diameter and the ovaries are producing adequate amounts of estradiol, another medication, human chorionic gonadotropin (hCG), is administered to get the eggs ready for fertilization.

The egg retrieval procedure is performed about thirty-six hours later. Once again, transvaginal ultrasound is used to visualize the ovarian follicles. Then an aspirating needle is placed through the vaginal wall into the ovary, and the follicular fluid along with the egg is aspirated from each follicle into a tube by applying suction. In this way, all the follicles in both ovaries are aspirated, and the eggs are collected. Once the eggs are obtained, they can be fertilized with a semen sample obtained from the woman's partner. Each of the eggs is placed in a separate petri dish together with a measured number of sperm cells, and the dishes are put into an incubator, where they develop into embryos, which can then be placed into the uterus of a gestational carrier. The carrier will have taken hormones to prepare her uterus to receive an embryo and to enable implantation to occur. The carrier is sometimes a relative of the woman whose baby she is carrying, sometimes a friend or even a volunteer not previously known to the couple. A legal agreement drawn up before pregnancy occurs will help avoid any legal difficulties in this process.

Embryo Freezing

In embryo freezing, eggs are obtained as described earlier, are fertilized and frozen using specialized techniques and equipment, and are subsequently thawed so they can be placed into a uterus. Embryos can be created and frozen before hysterectomy if timing and a woman's medical condition permit. At a future time, a woman can find a gestational carrier in whom the embryo or embryos can be implanted and may be carried through a pregnancy. The results of embryo freezing overall are not as successful as doing an egg retrieval and transferring the embryo to a uterus shortly after fertilization, but it does work well and may be seen as an option.

Egg Freezing

Similarly, in a few cases unfertilized eggs have been frozen and subsequently thawed and successfully fertilized and implanted in a carrier. This procedure is still experimental, but in the future, it might be attempted in a woman who needs oophorectomy at the time of hysterectomy and is not in a relationship with a partner. Once the eggs are frozen and the patient has a partner who can provide the sperm, the eggs can be thawed, fertilized, and implanted in a carrier or the embryo may be refrozen. A gestational carrier can be identified in the future, when the circumstances are more favorable to attempt pregnancy. We would like to emphasize that egg freezing and preservation are experimental and not available at this point as an option for women who anticipate ovarian removal.

Surrogacy

If your ovaries are removed at the time of hysterectomy, then neither your eggs nor your uterus will be able to be used to create an offspring. Another way to produce a family, *pure surrogacy*, involves finding a woman who is willing to be inseminated with your partner's sperm for the express purpose of becoming pregnant and carrying a pregnancy through delivery. The surrogate provides her own egg naturally for the pregnancy, and in vitro fertilization is not necessary. Again, we emphasize the importance of obtaining legal counsel and executing a legal agreement when undertaking these alternatives.

CHAPTER 13

Hormone Replacement Therapy

Whether she has a hysterectomy or not, every woman who lives to the age of menopause will confront the issue of hormone replacement. Hormone replacement therapy (HRT) has become one of the most discussed and debated issues related to women's health. The increased number of women encountering menopause as the baby boomer generation goes through middle age ensures that the discussion will continue and intensify. There are still many questions about the risks and benefits of hormone replacement, but a number of large studies are addressing those questions and perhaps will resolve controversies in coming years.

Women who have a hysterectomy and bilateral oophorectomy may need to address the issue of HRT somewhat earlier in their lives than most women. Women who have their uterus, but not their ovaries, removed face another dilemma—trying to figure out *when* they become menopausal, without the clue of monthly menstrual periods. Fortunately, a great deal of valuable information is available to help women with many of their questions and concerns.

Menopause occurs after a woman's last menstrual period. Since periods are apt to be irregular and widely spaced during perimenopause (the months and years preceding menopause), it can be hard to know exactly where you are. The wide age range (42 to 58) for menopause in healthy women indicates the wide variation in the number of eggs a woman has to begin with and their rate of loss.

Generally, when a woman has not had a period for a year, she is considered postmenopausal. At this point the ovaries have stopped ovulating for good because the ovarian follicles (the part of the ovary that contains the eggs) are depleted. When the ovarian follicles are depleted, the ovaries, which are the major source of the female sex hormones, stop producing hormones including estrogen and progesterone, both of which influence and are important for the functioning of many organ systems in the body.

When a woman goes through menopause naturally, it is a gradual and prolonged process. Her ovaries continue to produce small amounts of testosterone, a hormone that has a positive effect on sexual desire, for many years after menopause. However, when the ovaries are removed surgically, a significant source of testosterone production is removed, and surgical menopause causes a more rapid onset of symptoms that may be more extreme or more severe than with natural menopause.

SYMPTOMS OF MENOPAUSE

Eighty percent of women will experience hot flashes when they become menopausal. Other symptoms include night sweats, difficulty sleeping, memory loss, irritability, and mood changes. Later, most women will experience vaginal dryness. Sometimes urinary symptoms such as leakage, frequency, and urgency occur because of the loss of estrogen action on the urogenital tissues, which include the urethra and the supporting tissues around the bladder. Without estrogen these tissues may atrophy somewhat over time. The lack of ovarian hormones may also contribute to the development of osteoporosis, a gradual thinning of the bone that increases the risk of fractures. As estrogen decreases, blood lipids, especially cholesterol and LDL, increase. At one time it was thought that these changes contributed to the development of cardiovascular disease and that supplementation with estrogens in menopause would protect against heart disease. Recent data from large studies (WHI, HERS, which are discussed in the next section) have reversed this thinking and have demonstrated that estrogen replacement does not protect women from heart disease.

When both ovaries are removed surgically, there is a sudden loss of ovarian hormones—estrogen, progesterone, and, to a lesser extent, testosterone. Most women will notice an abrupt onset of hot flashes, difficulty sleeping, and night sweats. Often women are aware of memory changes, of feeling less sharp, and of having reduced sexual desire.

MAKING THE HRT DECISION

Whether to use hormone replacement therapy after hysterectomy is a personal decision that you should make in consultation with a medical professional who knows your full medical history and your concerns. Most women who start HRT after hysterectomy find that the hormones are beneficial in improving the immediate symptoms of menopause and in improving their sense of well-being.

Every woman has individual needs, but in general we recommend HRT for treatment of menopausal symptoms in women who

- have both ovaries removed at the time of hysterectomy;
- are already menopausal when they have a hysterectomy; and
- notice the development of menopausal signs and symptoms (hot flashes, night sweats, trouble sleeping, and so on) at any time after their hysterectomy, even if their ovaries have not been removed.

Initially, estrogen therapy will significantly reduce the number and frequency of hot flashes and other symptoms of menopause. You may not notice full effects until you have been on the medication for one month. We know from our patients and from the considerable research that has been done that many women feel that their quality of life is improved when they take estrogen. Estrogen therapy also has been shown to prevent bone loss and fractures.

In addition, estrogen therapy has been associated with other potential benefits such as a reduced risk of colon cancer, prevention of macular degeneration of the eye, and possible reduction in the development of Alzheimer disease. However, the jury is still out on whether estrogen protects against Alzheimer disease.

There are also risks associated with estrogen replacement alone. In women who have not had hysterectomies, one of the biggest risks is the development of endometrial cancer. That is why women who have *not* had hysterectomies and use HRT must take progesterone in some form along with the estrogen—progesterone has a preventive effect against endometrial cancer. Of course, if you have had a hysterectomy and no longer have a uterus, there is no risk of developing endometrial cancer and you can take estrogen alone. Estrogen therapy without progesterone is sometimes referred to as *unopposed estrogen* or estrogen replacement therapy (ERT).

A very small number of women develop clotting problems when they take estrogen. The risk of forming a blood clot in the lung (pulmonary embolus) or in the leg (venous thrombolism) is almost three times higher in women who take HRT than in women who don't take HRT, but this is still a tiny risk—about 3 in 10,000 women taking HRT get blood clots, compared with 1 in 10,000 women not taking HRT. Another possible risk of HRT is the worsening of gallstones, which could lead to the need for removal of the gallbladder. At this point, studies on the risk of breast cancer are inconclusive and contradictory, but there may be a very small increase in the risk of breast cancer after using HRT for ten years or longer. We discuss HRT and cancer in greater detail below.

Other side effects can include symptoms similar to what many women experience with their menstrual periods—bloating, breast tenderness, cramping, irritability, depression. A woman who has had a hysterectomy will not experience spotting or return of monthly periods. Usually dosage adjustments or changes in the way HRT is administered can address these problems.

Up until recently, ERT was thought to have many benefits including prevention of heart disease and strokes, improvement of cognitive function, and increased life expectancy. Except for the measurable positive effects on bone mass and the relief women experienced from acute menopausal symptoms such as hot flashes, vaginal dryness, and urinary tract dysfunction, the presumed advantages were based on simple comparisons between groups of women who had taken estrogen and those who had not. This type of observational study is subject to many variables or possibly biased influences and does not prove cause-and-effect relationships.

The most recent studies of HRT have many advantages and were designed to ask specific questions before women were even started on hormone treatment. Two trials were known as the Heart and Estrogen/ Progestin Replacement Study (HERS) and the Women's Health Initiative (WHI). HERS followed women with existing heart disease; WHI looked at healthy postmenopausal women to determine whether estrogens prevent heart disease and other chronic conditions. Both studies investigated a combination of conjugated equine estrogen (Premarin) and a synthetic progestin, medroxyprogesterone; the combination is called

Prempro. The studies found an early increase in heart problems and also found no protection from future cardiac disorders in users of HRT.

Shortly after the HERS study, the WHI study showed a slight increase in the risk of breast cancer. The comparative risks were equivalent to 30 cases/10,000 women among placebo (sugar pill) users and 38 cases/10,000 among those women taking Prempro. This translates to 8 more cases in 10,000 women (a risk of 0.08%), or less than one-tenth of 1 percent increased risk. Figures for other conditions are listed in table 13.1, which is based on 10,000 women taking Prempro for five years as compared with 10,000 women using the placebo.

The WHI study of the estrogen-progestin preparation was stopped at the end of five years because of the increase in incidence of breast cancer. The study was originally planned to last eight years. The results of the discontinued study apply *only* to Prempro users and not to users of other hormone replacement medications or schedules. Another group of women in the WHI study is still being followed; this group is taking estrogen alone (ERT), unaccompanied by a progesterone-like medication. This part of the study is of special interest to patients who have had a hysterectomy, because estrogen alone (again, referred to as unopposed estrogen or ERT) is the appropriate form of HRT following hysterectomy, as there is no need for a progestin to protect the endometrium of the uterus (but see below, about ovarian cancer).

If the estrogen alone (Premarin) group of the WHI turns out to show overall benefits, then the risks found in the Prempro trial may have been attributable to the progestin used in Prempro. Another recent observational study found that long-term use of unopposed estrogen may increase the risk of ovarian cancer. The ten-year risk was 1.8 times greater in women taking unopposed estrogen than in nonusers. But if at the time of hysterectomy a woman's ovaries are also removed, the chance of estrogen-induced abnormalities, including ovarian cancer, is virtually eliminated.

The bottom line is that estrogen should be taken with careful follow-up in *all* women, including those who have had a hysterectomy. Estrogen alone is safest for women who have had a hysterectomy, especially if the ovaries have also been removed. It should be taken primarily for the relief of postmenopausal symptoms and not indefinitely after menopause. Estrogens should be used to replace ovarian hormones in women who have had their ovaries removed prior to the anticipated normal

TABLE 13.1. RISKS WITH PREMPRO

	On HRT[a]	Not on HRT	Risk Ratio	Absolute Risk[b]
Heart attack	37	30	1.29	7/10,000
Stroke	29	21	1.41	8/10,000
Breast cancer	38	30	1.26	8/10,000
Colorectal cancer	10	16	0.66	6/10,000
Hip fracture	10	15	0.63	5/10,000

Source: Writing Group for the Women's Health Initiative Investigators, "Risks and Benefits of Estrogen plus Progestin in Healthy Postmenopausal Women: Principal Results from the Women's Health Initiative Randomized Controlled Trial," *JAMA* 288 (2002): 321–33.

[a] HRT = hormone replacement therapy.

[b] Absolute risk is the difference in number of cases for women not on HRT and women on HRT per 10,000 women per year.

menopause. Short-term use (up to two years beyond the menopausal age) is probably sufficient to eliminate menopausal symptoms. If severe symptoms persist, estrogen treatment should be continued to maintain a woman's quality of life.

GETTING STARTED

For women who wish to take estrogen replacement after surgery, we usually start them on ERT as soon after their surgery as possible. Unless your doctor believes there is a reason not to start, we recommend beginning ERT as soon as you are able to get out of bed, move around, and walk—a day or two after surgery.

If you still have your ovaries but are not having menstrual periods, it can be difficult to know when you reach menopause. Generally, when your ovarian hormonal function starts to wane, you will begin to experience the symptoms of menopause (hot flashes, etc.). In women who have had a hysterectomy, there is no disadvantage to starting hormone replacement as soon as symptoms suggestive of menopause begin. A blood test to determine follicle stimulating hormone (FSH) level can provide definitive information about the level of hormones being produced by your ovaries. If you are menopausal, your FSH level will be greater than 30 mIU/ml (milli International Units per milliliter), and your estradiol level will be less than 40 pg/ml (picograms per milliliter).

There is evidence that some women become menopausal at an earlier than expected age after they have had a hysterectomy, even though they retain their ovaries. As noted previously, this could be related to an alteration in the blood supply to the ovaries, which may occur as a result of the surgery.

Many types of estrogen in various forms are available for hormone replacement therapy. *Estradiol* is the active estrogen compound produced by the ovary. *Ethinyl estradiol* is a synthetic estrogen that has effects similar to those of estradiol. It is the same kind of estrogen used in oral contraceptives, but the dosage used for hormone replacement is about one-fourth to one-sixth that found in oral contraceptive pills. Conjugated estrogens are plant- or animal-based mixtures of various estrogens including estradiol and estrone, which is converted to estradiol in the body. Estrogens are available as pills that you take daily or transdermal patches that you apply to the skin twice weekly. Because different estrogens affect the body differently, the various forms of estrogen can be used to advantage to individualize therapy to best fit your personal needs. Your doctor will help you decide which forms would work best for you.

Women who have had a hysterectomy can usually take estrogen alone. Unlike menopausal women, who have an intact uterus and must also take a form of progesterone, women who have no uterus usually do not need to take additional hormones with estrogen as part of their HRT regimen. Progestins (the synthetic form of progesterone) are added to the HRT regimen of women with a uterus to counteract the growth effects of estrogen on the uterine lining. This growth can lead to endometrial cancer if estrogen is taken continuously without the addition of a progestin. Since your uterus has been removed, you do not have the added risk of endometrial cancer when you use estrogen alone.

Generally, hot flashes subside within three to four weeks after beginning HRT. You'll also notice an improved sense of well-being in about three weeks.

ALTERNATIVES TO HORMONE REPLACEMENT

Other medications may alleviate some the symptoms of menopause. None are as effective as estrogen in reducing hot flashes, however. These medications include *selective serotonin reuptake inhibitors* (SSRIs, often used to treat depression) or a progestin hormone based medication called *megestrol acetate* (Megace). Megace can reduce hot flashes but does have the side effect of promoting weight gain.

Another medication that is useful but not as effective as hormonal medications is *clonidine* (Catapres). Clonidine is used primarily to treat hypertension, but in some women it helps reduce hot flashes. It is usually administered in the form of a skin patch. Side effects can include dizziness or fatigue.

Some women find there are certain triggers, such as stress or alcohol, that set off their hot flashes, and avoiding these triggers can reduce the hot flashes. Caffeine can also be a trigger—for some women, drinking caffeinated beverages increases the number or severity of hot flashes, and limiting caffeine intake can be helpful.

If you choose not to or are unable to take estrogens, moderately effective alternative treatments for vaginal dryness are available. As noted earlier, vaginal lubricants are available over the counter and help increase moisture in the vagina. Vitamin E, applied to the vaginal area, may reduce vaginal discomfort. In addition, new products such as an estrogen-releasing vaginal ring (Estring) and a vaginal tablet (Vagifem) that releases tiny amounts of estrogen slowly are available. These products deliver small amounts of estrogen to the vagina and lead to minimal absorption of estrogen in the rest of the body. They are very effective in reducing vaginal discomfort. You will need a prescription for these estrogen products.

Many advocates of alternative medical approaches have publicized the use of soy products to alleviate menopausal symptoms. However, the few studies that have been done so far have shown that most of these soy preparations have little or no effect on symptoms of menopause in most women. But a diet rich in soy protein has been shown to reduce total cholesterol, LDL cholesterol, and triglycerides. And eating a diet containing large amounts of soy protein doesn't seem to have any adverse side effects.

Our information about phytoestrogens (plant estrogens), which are found in certain food sources, is incomplete. However, it is true that women who live in societies in which large amounts of phytoestrogens are consumed as part of the ordinary diet seem to have a lower incidence of some of the chronic diseases linked to estrogen deficiency. A word of caution is important. The use of any preparation that has the biological effects of estrogen, including "natural" products, may still share the adverse effects of estrogen.

A relatively new type of drug called *selective estrogen replacement modulators* (SERMs) offers a new approach to estrogen replacement therapy. Drugs in this category have been shown to increase bone mineral density in the hips and spine, as do estrogens, and to protect to some extent against cardiovascular disease. They do not have growth-promoting effects on the uterine lining and also appear to lack breast stimulatory properties. They may be valuable for women who do not wish to take or cannot take estrogens—for example, those with a history of breast cancer. One drawback of SERMs is that they may cause hot flashes rather than relieve them.

HRT and Cancer

A woman who has had uterine, cervical, or ovarian cancer or endometriosis may have concerns about HRT. Indeed, there is much we do not know about the effects of hormone replacement on different types of cancer.

Limited information is available about the use of estrogen therapy after treatment for endometrial or ovarian cancer. Some studies show that estrogen therapy used in conjunction with a progestin seems to be relatively safe in women who have been treated for early-stage endometrial cancer and who have been disease-free for at least a year after treatment. Your cancer specialist knows you and your situation in detail and is the best and most knowledgeable medical person to help you decide whether hormone replacement is an option for you.

With ovarian cancer, even less is known about the effects of hormone replacement therapy. Few studies regarding hormone replacement and ovarian cancer have been done. We know that the use of oral contraceptive medication for a moderate amount of time actually reduces the risk of ovarian cancer. However, a recent report suggests a relationship between estrogen use and mortality from ovarian cancer. If a relationship exists, it is very small.

Cervical cancer is a non-hormone-dependent cancer, and using hormone replacement therapy after treatment for cervical cancer does not seem to be a problem. If endometriosis is your problem, the decision about HRT is an individual one that you must make in consultation with your doctor. Since endometriosis seems to be influenced by hormones, especially estrogen, HRT may increases your risk for recurrent endometriosis. However, since many women who are treated for endometriosis with a hysterectomy and bilateral salpingo-oophorectomy are young, the overall benefits of hormone replacement may outweigh these risks of recurrence. And some 10 to 15 percent of women who have had hysterectomy and removal of both ovaries experience recurrence of endometriosis symptoms even when they do *not* use hormone replacement following the surgery.

There has been a great deal of publicity about the association between HRT and breast cancer, but there is a limited amount of data available and uncertainty about the relationship. Some research suggests that HRT might increase the risk of breast cancer or of recurrence in women who are breast cancer survivors. Other studies show reduced mortality in breast cancer survivors who use HRT. If you have had breast cancer or have a strong family history of the disease, your doctor might suggest remedies other than HRT for menopausal symptoms. But guidelines are not definitive—there are many factors to consider, such as the extent of disease and if it had spread to your lymph nodes and whether your cancer was positive for estrogen receptors. Again, your cancer specialist is the best person to advise you.

Each woman and her physician must consider priorities and establish a risk/benefit ratio based on the woman's specific benefits (osteoporosis prevention, relief from severe menopausal symptoms, and so on) and the risks in her particular situation.

Conclusion

eavy uterine bleeding, pelvic pain, or pelvic pressure may be symptoms of any of a number of gynecologic conditions. For nearly all these conditions, hysterectomy is one option for treatment, but, as we have discussed in this book, there are other options as well. In fact, there are only a few instances in which hysterectomy is done in an emergency situation (such as when a woman hemorrhages after childbirth) or as a lifesaving procedure (as a treatment for cancer, for example).

There are many reasons that a physician might recommend a hysterectomy to his or her patient, but as we have seen, generally this recommendation comes after other treatment options have been tried. And most of the time, hysterectomy is used as treatment of gynecologic conditions because the woman herself chooses it as definitive treatment for her symptoms. Sometimes this is an easy decision; other times it is not. We understand that deciding on surgery can be a difficult decision, and we generally recommend other treatments before we recommend surgery—and then only if the other treatments do not control the symptoms or if the other treatments produce intolerable side effects (as medications sometimes do).

A recent editorial in the *New England Journal of Medicine* was titled "Hysterectomy—Still a Useful Operation."* In this editorial, Drs. Joseph I. Schaffer and Ann Word summarize the results of a study involving 1,299 women, which showed that "88 percent of the women who had moderate to severe pelvic pain before surgery had significant improvement in this symptom" two years after surgery. It is because we

---

New England Journal of Medicine 347, no. 17 (2002): 1360–61.

have seen similar results with our own patients that we have written this book—not to "hype hysterectomy," but to educate women about the other treatments available to them as well as about the benefits of hysterectomy and when hysterectomy is the best treatment. Complete and up-to-date information helps any woman not only make the decision that is right for her but also feel confident about her decision.

Index